I0192615

SURVIVING
— YOUR —
HOSPITAL STAY

*A Nurse Educator's Guide to Staying
Safe and Living to Tell About It!*

JULIE SIEMERS, DNP, MSN, RN

Copyright © 2023

All rights reserved. All content is subject to copyright and may not be reproduced in any form without express written consent from the author. Although the author and publisher have made every effort to ensure that the information in this book was correct at press time, the author and publisher do not assume and hereby disclaim any liability to any party for any loss, damage, or disruption caused by errors or omissions, whether such errors or omissions result from negligence, accident, or any other cause.

Published by Elevate Publishing, Roswell, Georgia

ISBN 979-8-9862830-1-2 (paperback)

Printed in the United States of America

This book is dedicated to my loving parents, notably my mother, who said to me when I was 16 years old, "Why don't you become a nurse"? It has been one of the best decisions I've ever made. I became the nurse I am today because of their emotional and financial support, lifelong encouragement, and unwavering belief in me.

I want to thank each of my seven children for supporting me through the many years of studying and writing papers in between their dance lessons and soccer games. They missed days of playing at the park and weekend matinees to support my educational journey. They understood my passion and commitment to elevate the education of nurses in order to positively impact patient safety.

To anyone who may have suffered harm or loss because of the healthcare system, you have inspired me to take massive action to inform, educate, and create a positive impact on patient safety across the globe.

CONTENTS

This book contains the opinions of its author. It is intended to provide helpful and informative material on the subjects addressed in this publication. It is sold with the understanding that the author and publisher are not engaged in rendering medical, health, or another kind of personal professional services in this book. The reader should consult his or her medical, health or other competent professional before adopting any of these suggestions in this book or drawing inferences from it. The author and publisher specifically disclaim all responsibility for any liability, loss, or risk, personal or otherwise, that is incurred as a consequence, directly or indirectly, of the use and application of any of the contents of this book.

INTRODUCTION

The names of the patients whose lives we save can never be known. Our contribution will be what did not happen to them.

—Dr. Don Berwick, President & CEO of IHI, 2004.

Did you know that preventable medical error is the *third leading cause of death* in the United States? Are you aware that preventable medical error is both a national and international health crisis? Most individuals are completely unaware of the crisis of medical errors causing preventable patient deaths over the past several decades. More concerning is how many healthcare professionals are not even aware of the gravity of the situation and how many lives are impacted each year. "The healthcare delivery system is vulnerable to medical errors because of its decentralized and fragmented nature" (Bonney, 2014).

"The problem of patient safety has been repeatedly identified in mainstream news and the medical literature since the mid-1950s, but repeated revelations about patient deaths and injuries resulting from treatment have had almost no effect on the actual practice of medicine" (Millenson, 2002). Historically, the medical paradigm accepted in the United States is the belief that patient harm was part of the "risk of doing business." Not until very recently did some courageous healthcare professionals stop to question this deadly traditional paradigm.

In 1999, the Institute of Medicine (IOM) published a landmark study, "*To Err is Human*," estimating the occurrence of unnecessary and preventable patient deaths at between 44,000 and 98,000 annually. In response to this shocking report, U.S. President Bill Clinton called for mandatory reporting of medical errors and a drastic reduction in their prevalence. He also established a Center for Patient Safety at what's now known as Agency for Healthcare Research and Quality (AHRQ). *Mandatory reporting of medical errors never happened* and federal funds aimed at eradicating this issue have dried up.

Medical errors have been recognized in healthcare literature for over three decades, but have been severely underestimated. A literature review utilizing a tool to capture retrospective data estimated the annual number of preventable patient deaths in the U.S. to be between 250,000 and 400,000. This is a much higher incidence than the IOM reported in 1999 (Makary & Daniel, 2016; James, 2013). Why the discrepancy? The utilization of updated methods of retrieving and measuring tools in retrospective chart reviews were able to determine the harm experienced by patients more accurately.

Documenting patient safety events has always been challenging; safety metrics can be ill-defined and therefore difficult to measure and track. While the incidence of Healthcare Acquired Infections are fairly easy to identify, adverse drug events (patient harm resulting from medications) are not routinely tracked. Bates et al. (2023) report that the actual occurrence of adverse drug events occurs at nearly *20 times* the voluntary reporting system.

Not only do patients unnecessarily *die* from medical error, but many more patients experience some level of harm from interaction with the healthcare system—a system responsible for restoring or maintaining patients' health. James (2013) wrote in his article in the *Journal of Patient Safety*, reported that an additional four million to eight million patients are seriously injured each year from preventable medical errors. Some of these patients are so severely injured that they lose all quality of life. Many patients experience excruciating pain and discomfort as the result of a medical error. Countless patients linger in broken and dysfunctional bodies; some suffer and take years to die.

The shocking revelation of preventable patient deaths identified and published in *To Err is Human* (1999) launched the genesis of awareness in the healthcare community of these tragic occurrences. By highlighting and quantifying the devastating statistics of preventable patient deaths due to medical error in this landmark report, the IOM has personalized the data, making it meaningful to the average person who may become a patient. Healthcare communities have not been forthcoming with this information, nor have they shared these appalling statistics with patients and their families.

These devastating events have been a dirty little secret that has been silenced with monetary payoffs to families (with or without litigation) or swept under the proverbial rug. In 2023, we live in the Information Digital Age where patients and their families now have access to crucial information literally at their fingertips. Healthcare consumers must take the opportunity to become informed and educated, paving the way for a partnership with nurses and physicians to change the current trajectory of preventable patient harm and death. It's time for radical transparency across all levels of our healthcare system to eradicate the meaningless deaths of so many human beings.

A Global Problem

Unfortunately, the problem of preventable medical errors in healthcare settings is not unique to the U.S. Globally, multiple countries report statistics of preventable patient deaths in their healthcare systems. Nearly 1 in 10 patients admitted into health-care facilities experience an adverse event (de Vires et al., 2008, Panagioti et al., 2019). In 2015, the UK estimated over 1000 avoid-able deaths per month were occurring in their hospitals (Waldie et al., 2016). Canada also ranks preventable medical error as the third leading cause of death where one of 18 hospital visits result in preventable harm. The Canadian Patient Safety Institute reports statistics of patient harm comparative to the U.S., stating "In our healthcare system, there is a death from patient harm every 13 minutes and 14 seconds." The cost of healthcare treat-ment incurred from preventable medical errors is estimated at $2.75 billion every year (www.patientsafetyinstitute.ca).

The World Health Organization, European office, reported medical errors and related adverse events occur in 8% to 12% of hospitalizations. The Quality in Australian Health Care Study found that almost 17% of patients hospitalized suffered an adverse event (Millenson, 2002). The United Kingdom, Spain, France, and Denmark have published data with similar adverse events statistics, demonstrating patient safety is a global issue (https://www.euro.who.int/en/health-topics/Health-systems/patient-safety/data-and-statistics).

Here are some shocking statistics to contemplate: You are more likely to die of a medical error in the hospital than be killed in an airplane crash, a bomb, or a mass shooting. If the esti-mated minimum number of 250,000 preventable patient deaths per year, or 685 patients per day and over 28 patients dying every hour is applied to the following the examples, here is what that may look like:

Boeing's 747 airplane has the capacity to hold 467 passen-gers. 250,000 patients dying a preventable death each year is equivalent to 1.1 airplanes falling out of the sky and all passen-gers aboard perishing *every single day*. Would that be a headline that would create panic, anger, and a march against the airline industry if this truly happened? Yet this is what is happening in healthcare across the globe. Yankee stadium holds 54,000 people. 250,000 patient deaths in the hospital would be equivalent to 4.6 stadiums full of people dying if a bomb went off and killed everyone in Yankee Stadium. How is it that this catastrophic number of patients being harmed and dying has not impacted a massive movement of change in healthcare safety? The outcry from families of patients having suffered harm and death from incompetent medical care and errors have not been heard loud enough.

Why hasn't the healthcare system changed and adopted accountability measures from organizations and healthcare providers? Why does public outrage dissipate over time and national media coverage fade away? Without constant pressure and fighting for change in our healthcare systems, policy revisions and adopting safety practices will not occur. Individuals joining together to create a public outcry is essential to create a sustainable transformation for patient safety. Healthcare providers are *obligated* by the professional code of ethics to do well and prevent any harm when providing care for patients (Ghazal et al., 2014).

Every patient deserves and has the right to expect and experience safe healthcare. Every patient should be able to trust that they will be well cared for and won't experience harm; their health and safety should not be endangered when interacting with the healthcare system. Both nurses and physicians are expected to operate within industry guidelines and standards of care when interacting within the healthcare system and caring for patients. These national care guidelines, *standards of care*, are utilized by attorneys in medical legal cases to determine potential negligence when a patient experiences harm or death in the healthcare system. Why does it take a court of law to uphold these standards and expectations in some cases?

According to the Center for Medicare and Medicaid Services, healthcare safety has declined since the COVID-19 pandemic in 2020 (Fleisher et al., 2022). Patient safety has been a well-known challenge and discussion in healthcare arenas for the past several decades; ironically, this global problem is not one that most patients or their families are even aware of (Sutton et al., 2023). Now is the time to become informed and take an active role in your own health and that of your loved ones.

It is deplorable that medical errors occur and have taken such a catastrophic toll on thousands of families. I anticipate that this book may cause a great stir of uncomfortable feelings in both the medical profession, nursing profession and healthcare in general. It may even create some angry comments or an outcry of denial and finger-pointing. But change *must* occur. The healthcare community must adopt radical transparency at large; this enormous and far-reaching problem may touch every human being on the planet.

This book was written with the intent to empower you with a basic knowledge of what to expect in the hospital and how you can mitigate harm; you must take your health into your own hands. The time has arrived for patients, their families and loved ones to take charge of their own healthcare. You cannot leave this to chance or hope. You must be an active participant in your health with awareness and the courage to create a plan for a healthy and safe journey. This may mean a paradigm shift in which *you* will take back the power for your personal well-being that you have inadvertently given to healthcare providers.

As someone actively engaged in the healthcare system for over four decades, I want to share my experience and knowledge to help you on your journey through the medical environment. We will discuss information and concepts commonly experienced by patients and what you should expect. With your new awareness and knowledge, my hope is that you will gain confidence and feel more comfortable and empowered to navigate the healthcare experience.

This book has been "under construction" for quite a few years; I can no longer ignore the call I feel deep in my heart to share this with you. I hope this will empower you to advocate for yourself and your loved ones. If just *one* life is saved from an unexpected injury or preventable death by something you learn in these pages, my purpose will have been fulfilled and my heart will sing. Keep reading to understand how you can be an active participant and advocate for the safety of your health and that of your loved ones.

IT'S HARD TO KILL A HEALTHY 15-YEAR-OLD

The Story of Lewis Blackman

Lewis Blackman, a healthy, gifted 15-year-old boy, tragically lost his life due to a multitude of medical errors by both nurses and physicians. Lewis underwent elective surgery on his chest deformity that he was born with, pectus excavatum, at the Medical University of South Carolina, a teaching hospital with a good reputation and modern equipment. Lewis and his parents believed this to be a very safe surgery; the hospital and the surgeons had a good reputation. They believed they were in good hands; they believed Lewis would be taken care of. His nurses and physicians, every single one of them, missed the signs that Lewis was becoming unstable over many hours and was in grave danger. He lost the battle for his life when he bled to death over a 30-hour period, despite copious evidence of alarming clinical decline. *Each of those hours presented an opportunity for a nurse, a resident, or a physician to evaluate the physiological deterioration that was taking place before their eyes.* Nobody was looking; every eye was blind to Lewis's perilous condition—except for Lewis's mother's—but tragically, nobody listened to her.

After surgery in the recovery room, the surgeon told Lewis's parents that the surgery went well. The medical chart noted that Lewis wasn't making much urine; his intravenous fluids were inadequate. Lewis was given a medication for his pain, Toradol (Ketorolac), a medication that can have many harmful side effects. Toradol is not approved for use in most of Europe but is widely used in the U.S. *The guidelines for this medication state that it shouldn't be given in low urine output states; dangerous risks of this medication are internal bleeding and perforated ulcers.*

Saturday evening, several days after surgery, Lewis begins to run a slight fever and his feet are cold to the touch. *Cold extremities indicate poor perfusion, a warning sign that the body is shunting or saving blood for the vital organs, a sign of shock.* Lewis continues to receive Toradol for the pain.

On Sunday morning, Lewis complains of abdominal pain to his mother, stating "It's the worst pain imaginable." Lewis's mother (Helen) reports this to the nurse who states that it is "gas pain" and "There is nothing I can do for gas pain" and suggests he needs to move around. Another nurse suggests a bath for Lewis; his mother reports that he "is getting weaker and weaker." The nurses then suggest that Lewis needs to walk in the halls, even though Lewis complains that his pain is getting worse (as he is still receiving Toradol).

By Sunday afternoon the pain continues. Lewis's abdomen is firm and distended, *a sign that something is definitely wrong!* His skin is pale and cool, his temperature has dropped and he's dripping with cold sweat. His eyes are sunken, he's exhausted, and is in constant pain at this point. Helen repeatedly voices her concerns to the nurses and requests that a veteran physician evaluate her son. Her imploring appeals are all but ignored; she knows something is desperately wrong with her son.

Sunday evening, the chief resident finally comes to evaluate Lewis and orders a suppository for a "blocked intestine." *A resident is an apprentice doctor; though licensed, they don't have the judgment or experience of a veteran doctor.* Lewis's mother does not realize this man is not a veteran doctor. In his evaluation note, the chief resident writes Lewis's heart rate is "~80s" (*was he guessing because he forgot to measure?*), while a nurse documents at the same time in another part of the chart that Lewis's heart is beating at 126 times per minute. (*She had just measured the heart rate, presenting a huge discrepancy in documentation. A heart rate of 126 is a sure sign of distress.*) The chief resident reassures Helen that the "sweating" is a side-effect of the medication. By this time, Lewis has had zero urine output for over 12 hours (*this should have alerted the nurses and doctors to a serious problem*). By midnight, Lewis's heart rate has increased to 142 beats per minute and his temperature has dropped to 95 degrees Fahrenheit. *That these vital signs do not cause alarm bells to be ringing louder than a three-alarm fire to signal the impending catastrophe is frankly egregious and unbelievable.*

Somehow, Lewis survives the night and on Monday morning, his pain suddenly stops. Lewis now has gone 24 hours with no urine output. The nurses cannot detect a blood pressure but believe the machine to be broken; the nurses attempt 12 times to obtain a blood pressure unsuccessfully over the next two hours. Still, no one calls a veteran physician. Lewis's mother asks the resident why her son's lips are pale and the same color as his skin. "Oh, that's just that low blood pressure. It pulls the blood away from the capillaries to protect the vital organs." *Yes, sir, this is a classic sign of shock and requires immediate action to save the patient's life! How were the signs of shock and of patient deterioration missed by so many medically trained individuals?*

Lewis's mother notices Lewis trying to say something, but his speech is slurred; his mother finally hears him say, "It's going black." Lewis's mother calls for help and finally, a Code 99 (Code Blue) is called; it is chaotic, with over 20 team members responding. They are shocked and can't understand why Lewis is in cardiac arrest; they had told each other he was getting better.

Surgeons rush in, ask Helen to leave the room, and proceed for over an hour to try to revive Lewis and bring him back to life. They are too late; much too late.

Lewis's mother initially refused an autopsy, but agreed when her husband encouraged it after the physicians stated, "We don't know what went wrong, we don't know what happened." Upon autopsy, nearly 3 liters of blood was found in Lewis's abdomen; a normal amount of blood in the whole body of a person Lewis's size is between 4–5 liters. His severe abdominal pain was from a perforated ulcer, a deadly side-effect of Toradol. Egregious misses by both nurses and medical residents occurred during these last days of Lewis's life. Assumptions were made. This was a healthy child coming in for elective surgery. Their minds were not set to receive the idea of a complication, and Helen's worries didn't penetrate.

Permission for publication by Helen Haskell, mother of beloved Lewis Blackman.

KEY TAKEAWAYS

- Trust your intuition when you feel something is wrong.
- Understand normal vital sign ranges (discussed in Chapter 10).
- Ask questions and keep asking questions.
- Unusual or unexpected levels of pain should be further investigated.
- Escalate your concerns to the hospital House Supervisor and Chief Medical Officer if necessary.
- Give yourself grace in "not knowing" enough about healthcare.

CHAPTER 2

MEDICAL ERRORS
Shocking and Inconceivable!

Medical error is defined as the unintentional act of harming a patient or an act that does not achieve its intended outcome. A medical error can result from either the error of execution, an error in planning or "use of a wrong plan to achieve an aim" (Martinez et al., 2017). Most medical errors do not occur because of the incompetence or negligence of an individual healthcare provider. Both human error at the individual caregiver level (nurse, doctor, physical therapist, etc.) and broken systems within healthcare organizations contribute to most preventable medical errors.

The Agency of Healthcare Research and Quality (AHRQ) reports that medical errors are frequently caused by "human problems" such as not adhering to policy, procedures, and guidelines for patient safety (Van den Bos et al., 2015). Poor communication systems, cognitive bias influencing crucial decisions and actions, distractions, and fatigue can contribute to the breakdown in safe patient care delivery (Bonney, 2014; Sorrel, 2017).

All medical errors are not the result of malpractice; malpractice involves negligence or incompetence by a healthcare provider that results in patient harm. If the healthcare provider is reckless, careless, or fails to provide adequate and appropriate care to the patient as per "standards of care" guidelines, patients may experience harm or death. (Bonney, 2014).

Typically, medical errors are categorized by "what happened" to cause the harm or death to the patient, such as a medication error, a diagnostic error or a healthcare acquired infection (HAI). Preventable medical error may result in short-term or long-term physical harm or may even be the cause of a patient's untimely death. Any of these adverse outcomes can be catastrophic to patients and their families. Preventable medical error that causes injury, harm, or death to a patient may be caused by either a healthcare provider doing something "wrong" or failing to do what is expected in the circumstance.

According to the study from Daniel R. Levinson, inspector general of the Department of Health and Human Services, "Hospitals are to track medical errors and adverse patient events, analyze their causes and improve care." In Mr. Levinson's report he stated, "Despite the existence of incident reporting systems, *hospital staff did not report most events that harmed Medicare beneficiaries*" (https://liferaftgroup.org/2012/04/new-report-finds-most-hospital-errors-go-unreported/).

In a *New York Times* article, "Report Finds Most Errors at Hospitals Go Unreported," Robert Pear (2012) explained that federal investigators have shown that hospital employees recognize and report only one out of seven errors, accidents and other events that harm Medicare patients while they are hospitalized. Out of 293 cases of patient harm found by federal investigators, only five led to a change in policy or procedure. This is abysmal and so disappointing.

The lack of transparency and accountability means that mistakes are rarely identified and investigated. Mistakes and errors should be monitored and analyzed to prevent future occurrences. It is imperative that analysis and learning occurs in a healthy environment of support within healthcare systems; it is essential to mitigate errors and prevent future safety events. Patient outcomes should be transparent; reporting of harmful events and "near misses" should be mandatory. How do we improve patient safety if mistakes are hidden away, secretive, and not discussed or shared? The goal of healthcare should be to bring the patient back to a state of health as effectively and quickly as possible; the quality of life for each patient should be maximized to the individual's level of health.

The Patient Safety Overview (2021) reports that at least 50% of hospitalized patients' harm could be prevented. If there has been negligible improvement in patient harm over the past fifteen years (Ahsani-Esthbanati et al., 2022), could the lack of reporting be contributing to this global calamity? By treating errors and mistakes as secrets and failing to disclose and discuss the situation, patient safety will continue to be a leading cause of preventable death.

To clarify, there is a difference between a patient dying in the hospital from a medical condition that deteriorates and a preventable medical error. "All bad results are not negligence; sometimes the disease wins" (Schlachter, 2017). There are times that a patient's disease process will cause the deterioration of the physical body; these events may be unavoidable and are not the blame or failure of a person or even the healthcare system. For example, physicians cannot prevent the extension of a bleed in the brain or a stroke if a blood vessel is weak and it tears or ruptures. The blood may leak out of the vessel and accumulate in the tissue, causing severe neurological problems or even death. This is something that is out of the healthcare team's control. "Sometimes a patient's body does something unexpected, and despite the efforts of alert and competent practitioners, the patient gets sicker or dies. Due to the complexity of variables present during surgery, some patients may die during the procedure without an error or evidence of malpractice occurring (Schlachter, 2017).

"Failing to plan" may be considered a medical error if healthcare providers are not thorough in preparing for procedures or surgery. If a physician fails to review a diagnostic test (such as an MRI) when planning an intricate surgery, they may encounter and be unprepared for a thinning or fragile blood vessel during the surgery. The lack of planning and preparing can be disastrous. It is risky to operate near a fragile blood vessel as it may rupture and cause the patient to hemorrhage. Unfortunately, the patient and their family cannot know what really happened in these types of situations unless they know what to look for in the medical record. The documentation may even be missing or may be poorly communicated in the medical record.

Acts of Commission or Omission

Joe (pseudonym), a 34-year-old patient, was admitted to the hospital for spinal surgery to repair a herniated disc in his back. Post-surgery, Joe was given a Patient Controlled Analgesia (PCA) or "pain pump" programmed with a specific dose of morphine ordered by the doctor. The PCA pump is designed for the patient to give themselves a prescribed dose of pain medication when they feel pain. Opioid medications such as morphine, are commonly prescribed pain medications to be delivered through a PCA pump. The most concerning and life-threatening side-effect of an opioid is a slowing of the breathing rate, or respiratory depression.

It is expected and essential for the nurse or healthcare team to monitor the patient's vital signs closely, primarily the respiratory rate, for a patient receiving an opioid through a PCA pump. The patient's breathing rate is vital to life and must be monitored closely; a slowing of the patient's breathing rate can result in apnea or "no breathing." If not observed and addressed, the patient can ultimately stop breathing, leading to injury or death.

Other crucial assessment points include measuring the oxygen saturation, the patient's level of consciousness, heart rate and blood pressure. Joe was not monitored as closely or as often as he should have been; nobody noticed that Joe's breathing had slowed significantly until he just stopped breathing completely.

When the nurse found him unresponsive and called a Code Blue, it was too late; they couldn't resuscitate him. Joe's preventable death was another tragic statistic of an unnecessary death. The nurse later admitted she didn't monitor him closely and was "shocked" that he was dead; she stated she "got busy" caring for her other patients. As she was planning care and her tasks for her shift, she deemed Joe as a stable patient in the "low risk" category who therefore didn't require close surveillance. She assumed he should have been a stable patient; his young age and lack of other health problems deemed him "low risk" for complications in her mind. The nurse omitted accurately assessing Joe; she did not exercise vigilance in caring for him. She did not monitor Joe's respiratory rate, level of consciousness or neurological status, or other pertinent vital signs. We will talk further about vital signs and medications in future chapters.

The National Patient Safety Foundation (NPSF) is a non-profit organization with a vision and goal to help hospitals attain the goal of ZERO preventable patient injuries and deaths due to healthcare errors. The NPSF describes two main categories of error—those that occur primarily from an act of *commission*, a wrong action taken (or an incorrect treatment), or an act of *omission*, action not taken (failure to diagnose or treat), or something not done that should have been (Rodziewicz et al., 2020; Bates et al., 2023).

Joe's story is an example of an act of omission; he did not get the care he needed to survive. An act of omission occurs when an expected action by a healthcare provider, based on *standards of care* or medical training, does not occur. When nursing care is omitted or forgotten, or a nurse misses a step in a process, patient harm can occur (Mushta et al., 2018). Nursing care that is "left undone" or "unfinished" may contribute to poor patient outcomes and is estimated to occur 55% to 98% in expected nursing care (Labrague et al., 2021). These errors of omission in patient care can lead to a temporary impairment of the patient's health, a long-term impairment, permanent impairment, or death.

The length of stay for the patient for a particular diagnosis is the average time a patient should need acute care or close monitoring. If an act of omission or commission occurs, it may lead to a longer length of stay for a patient, resulting in poor outcomes and a significant financial burden for the hospital. These events are frequently not reimbursed by insurance companies or Medicare and Medicaid. Studies have identified that a high proportion of errors of omission manifest most prominently as failure to follow accepted management pathways for common clinical conditions.

An example of an act of commission type of error is "wrong site surgery" and "wrong patient surgery." Wrong-site surgery has been one of the top three sentinel events cited by the Joint Commission for several decades, impacting nearly 40 patients each week (Patra, 2022)! For example, a wrong-site surgery is when the physician and surgical team mistakenly remove the healthy and functioning kidney rather than the diseased and non-functioning kidney, leaving it still inside the patient. Unfortunately, despite widespread prevention measures implemented in 2004, these horrific errors still occur today.

Other surgically related errors reported in the literature and anecdotally have been foreign bodies such as surgical sponges and instruments accidentally left inside the patient's body, causing infection and intense pain for the patient. Surgeries can and do go wrong. Dimova et al. (2018) reports of a surgeon accidentally puncturing the dura mater, the tough protective membrane covering the brain and spinal cord, causing the cerebrospinal fluid to leak out of the enclosed area, causing patient harm.

Medication errors are another example of an act of commission. In 1995, the *Boston Globe* ran this headline: "Doctor's order killed cancer patient." Dana Farber Cancer Center was a prominent institution supposedly delivering quality care to its patients with cancer. On this fateful day, a physician's prescribed order resulted in the administration of a lethal dose of chemotherapy, killing a 39-year-old patient being treated for breast cancer. Her mother wrote a chilling letter to the Patient Safety Conference in June of 2000, appealing to the members to pause and think about the many patients who are gone now due to a medical error; how many patients were harmed by a healthcare system that was supposed to help them, to heal them? She implored them to acknowledge the fact that patient safety must be constant and ingrained in the system and into caring hearts.

A 75-year-old woman died several years ago at a major hospital in the Midwest; she was mistakenly given a paralyzing medication instead of a sedative medication (see story in Chapter 15). Reports indicate several of the safety protocols for administering medications were bypassed by the nurse, resulting in a loss of life. A family lost a wife and a mother on that fateful day (https://www.tennessean.com/story/money/2018/12/04/vanderbilt-hospital-death-vumc-nurse-error-patient/2204869002/).

Healthcare providers are tasked with the primary responsibility to provide safe care to patients and to restore the patient to their optimum health. Nurses are one of the most essential elements and key personnel responsible in helping to prevent medical errors. Of all healthcare providers, nurses are the front-line care givers and spend the most time at the patient's bedside. Nurses are responsible for "continuity in patient care and follow-up; they are primarily responsible for the protection and development of health" (Seyma et al., 2021). Later in this book we will discuss the multiple tasks and duties nurses have and how you can support and assist them in caring for your family or loved ones.

KEY TAKEAWAYS

- Medical errors and adverse events are grossly underreported.
- At least 50% of hospitalized patients' harm could be prevented.
- An act of *commission* is a wrong action taken, or an incorrect treatment given.
- An act of *omission* is an action not taken or failure to do something that should have been done.
- ZERO patient harm is what patients should expect and deserve.
- Patients should be safe in the healthcare system.

CHAPTER 3

SAFETY IN HEALTHCARE
Why is Healthcare Downright Dangerous?

The Institute of Medicine (IOM) has defined and modified the definition of safety in its publications over the past few decades. These definitions will be helpful for you to understand as we dive deeper into this topic throughout the book:

- Safety—the "freedom from accidental injury" (1999)
- Safe care—"avoiding injuries to patients from the care that is intended to help them" (2001)
- Error—failures of planned actions to be completed as intended, or the use of wrong plans to achieve what is intended (2004)
- Adverse events—injuries caused by medical intervention (2004)
- Preventable medical error—an adverse event that is the result of an error (2004)

The idea of a safety culture in American hospitals has been recognized and discussed in the healthcare literature, and at conferences and forums for decades. In 2019, the Agency for Healthcare Research and Quality (AHRQ) cited two studies which attempted to understand harm caused by healthcare. In the California study in 1978 by Don Harper Mills, the goal was "to obtain adequate information about patient disabilities resulting from health care management." In the second study in 1984, Harvard Medical Practice studied adverse patient outcomes during health care delivery. Both large-scale studies concluded there was an enormous problem in the frequency and impact of medical errors. Unfortunately, neither study resulted in significant changes in medical practice.

Subsequent studies have found the annual rate of patients experiencing harm in the hospital average between 10–12%; almost half of these occurrences were deemed preventable. "The problem of patient safety has been repeatedly identified in the medical literature since the mid-1950s, but regular revelations about patient deaths and injuries resulting from treatment have had almost no effect on the actual practice of medicine" (Millenson, 2002).

Healthcare organizations are well aware of the continued occurrences of preventable medical error within their walls. Implementation of strategies thought to decrease patient harm have been adopted at various institutions; a few were found to be partially successful. Suggested solutions found in the literature to help hospitals focus on harm prevention:

- Address root cause
- Make designs of equipment, systems, and processes more intuitive
- Make wrong actions more difficult
- Make incorrect actions correct
- Make it easier to discover error

The Lucian Leape Institute identified key elements for making healthcare safer (https://www.ihi.org/Engage/Initiatives/Lucian-Leape-Institute/Pages/default.aspx):

- Transparency
- Patient/consumer engagement
- Restoration of joy and meaning in work and workforce safety
- Care integration
- Medical education reform

Unfortunately, very few changes to healthcare practices have been implemented in medical practice over the past few decades. *Telling people to be more careful doesn't work.* Patient harm and patient deaths continue to occur multiple times a day across our country and globally. In 2016, researchers at Johns Hopkins University extrapolated data from hospital admissions and death rates from medical errors. This study concluded that 9.5% of all patients admitted to the hospital died from medical error (Sipherd, 2018).

Preventable medical error causes millions of patients annually to experience harm in the healthcare system (Andel et al., 2012). "Preventable safety events now occur in 115 of every 1,000 hospitalizations" with many of these patients reporting long-lasting effects from the medical error, leading to a loss of trust in the healthcare system. Approximately 400,000 patients each year experience some level of preventable harm in the healthcare system each year, costing billions of dollars annually (Rodziewicz et al., 2022). The patient death rate due to preventable medical harm remains staggering.

In searching for solutions to safety events, healthcare leaders have observed successful approaches in other high-risk industries. The aviation industry is fraught with risk and has multiple operation points for potential catastrophic error and outcomes. When student pilots were trained to fly simulators before they got in the actual cockpit, the training directly correlated to a decrease in flight errors and resulted in increased safety for the passengers. Healthcare leaders witnessed the effectiveness of this model of training and improved outcomes; this led to the adoption of simulation practice for nurses and doctors.

Pilots have been using a pre-flight checklist in the cockpit prior to lift-off to mitigate potential errors for decades. Surgeons in hospitals have now followed suit and recently adopted a pre-surgical checklist to prevent errors in the operating rooms. Studies have shown improvements in patient safety and preventing adverse events and medical errors with the adoption of checklists (Harris et al., 2020). Many positive patient outcomes have already been impacted by this proactive and preventative measure.

Hospitals need to be held accountable to implementing cultures of safety and creating safe environments for patients. Healthcare is tasked with restoring patients to their baseline health or better and returning home without harm or injury. Medical errors are costly at best and can tragically cause permanent harm or death at worst. As our healthcare system struggles to stay solvent, there is ample opportunity to provide safe patient care and decrease overall healthcare costs; it is a win-win opportunity for everyone.

Adverse Events

An adverse event is unintended physical harm or injury to a patient caused by medical care and healthcare management. Adverse events can cause an injury that prolongs hospitalization, produces a new patient disability, or may result in the patient's death. In addition to the 13.5% occurrence of temporary harm events, another 13.5% of Medicare patients experienced an adverse event during their hospital stay. The annual cost of medical errors is astronomical and estimated at costing between $17 billion and $20 billion (Van Den Bos et al., 2015; Andel et al., 2012; Rodziewicz et al., 2022).

Adverse events can be classified by the severity and impact on patients: significant serious, life-threatening, or fatal. As cited in a recent study, researchers found that larger hospitals had a higher incidence of adverse events as compared to smaller hospitals: adverse drug events accounted for 39% of errors and events associated with surgery or procedures accounted for 30% of the documented errors (Bates et al., 2023).

Adverse events can be classified as either preventable or nonpreventable. Preventable or avoidable events occur when rendered care did not meet the minimum standard of expected care, resulting in patient injury. An egregious example of substandard care occurred when a physician ordered feedings to be given to a patient through a tube in her abdomen. This tube was not a feeding tube; it was a tube for kidney dialysis. This disastrous mistake caused the patient pain, infection, and multiple organ dysfunction.

Nonpreventable adverse events may occur when the standards of expected care were met but the patient experiences an unavoidable negative outcome. An example of a nonpreventable adverse event occurred when a patient had an angiography to view his coronary arteries and suffered a stroke. During the procedure, a piece of plaque from the artery wall broke off and migrated to the patient's brain. This event was not due to the physician's negligence or an error; it is cited as one of the risks of this type of procedure and may be an unfortunate complication.

Temporary Harm Events

These events do not cause lasting harm but require intervention from the healthcare team. Reports indicate that 13.5% of Medicare patients receiving hospital care in 2008 experienced temporary harm and injury (Levinson, 2010). These statistics only capture some of the patients harmed—they do not account for the thousands of patients harmed each year that are not covered or tracked by Medicare. Federal regulations require hospitals participating in Medicare programs to "track medical errors and adverse patient events, analyze their causes, and implement preventative actions." Where can this information and data be found? Who is tracking it and who analyzes this data? What strategies have been implemented based on the analyzed data? These are questions that are not easily answered.

Near Miss

A near miss is an error committed by a healthcare provider, either by acting or failing to take appropriate action, which does not result in harm to the patient. The patient did not suffer any harm due to the early detection or by luck; it was a "close call" (Dimova et al., 2018). Near misses can happen for various reasons and may occur more frequently if the healthcare provider is distracted or not paying close attention to what she/he is doing. In 2001, the Joint Commission began requiring hospitals to report patient injuries due to near misses and medical errors. By compiling healthcare organizational patient harm events, the patterns or hazards should be communicated across healthcare networks as precautions and warnings to prevent similar harm to other patients.

Never Events

The term *"never event"* was first introduced in 2001 by Ken Kizer, MD, former CEO of the National Quality Forum (NQF). Dr. Kizer noted particularly shocking preventable medical errors that are 100% preventable and should never occur in the healthcare setting. An initial *never event* list was developed in 2002 because of further observations of egregious mistakes. Millenson (2002), cites several examples of these:

- Wrong-site surgery or wrong patient surgery. In Michigan, a surgeon removed the wrong breast when performing a mastectomy on a 69-year-old patient.

- A respiratory ventilator was mistakenly disconnected from a 73-year-old patient; she was unable to breathe without this machine and died.
- Objects left inside the body during surgery (surgical instruments or sponges).
- Transfusion of unmatched blood into a patient.
- Serious pressure ulcers are devastating to the patient and are very costly to the healthcare system; pressure ulcers are preventable and should never happen.

In 2008, the Centers for Medicare and Medicaid Services (CMS) adopted the term *"never events"* and disseminated a list; they refuse to compensate hospitals for additional patient care costs incurred due to a *never event*. The untold devastation to patients is appalling; over 400,000 *never events* were estimated to cost over $3.7 billion.

The list of *never events* has been revised multiple times, expanding to include preventable adverse events that are clearly identifiable, measurable, and serious, resulting in death or significant disability. The list now consists of 29 "serious reportable events" grouped into 7 categories by the AHRQ Patient Safety Network (PSNET):

- Surgical or procedural events
- Product or device events
- Patient protection events
- Care management events
- Environmental events
- Radiologic events
- Criminal events

Never events are egregious in the most serious sense of the word. If *never events* are preventable and healthcare systems are on high alert for these mishaps, why are they still occurring?

Sentinel Events

The Joint Commission defines a sentinel event as "a patient safety event that results in death, permanent harm or severe temporary harm." A sentinel event signals the need for an immediate investigation into the circumstances and outcome of the event. Often, a *never event* is also a sentinel event as just discussed:

- Surgery on the wrong individual or wrong body part
- Blood transfusion errors
- Retained foreign body after surgery
- Delay in treatment with poor patient outcomes
- Medication errors resulting in patient death
- Infant harm or death during delivery
- Bed rail-related entrapment death
- Look-alike, sound-alike drug names

The Joint Commission publishes newsletters highlighting the occurrence of these events to alert healthcare organizations and provide recommendations to reduce risk and prevent future occurrences. Although it is not mandatory to report a sentinel event to the Joint Commission, it is highly encouraged to raise awareness and prevent future patient harm.

Root cause analysis is a process utilized by organizations to determine where the system failed to keep the patient safe or when the individual healthcare provider made an error. Healthcare leaders are expected to review the occurrence of sentinel events to reduce harm to patients and to implement safeguards preventing future errors. The goal is zero events of patient harm—*no* patient should be harmed.

Most safety issues leading to patient harm are correctable. At a prominent hospital in New York, a strategic plan to reduce sentinel events was developed and implemented; after seven years of focused efforts, they reported an increase in positive patient outcomes. This team saw the rate of sentinel-events occurrence per 1,000 baby deliveries drop from 1.04 in the year 2000 to zero in 2008 and 2009. That is one baby dying for every thousand and now there are zero babies dying due to these focused efforts. The decrease in sentinel events equated to dropping payouts of more than $50 million down to $250,000 (Cohen, 2014). More important than the cost savings, of course, is the drastically improved quality of patient care and reduction of medical errors. Lives are saved when the medical profession prioritizes patient safety issues.

It is the expectation that when patients seek and receive healthcare, their condition or health improves. In 2001, the Institute of Medicine (IOM) released the paper *"Crossing the quality chasm"*; this paper spoke to the care Americans *should* be receiving and care they *were* receiving. The observed and reported data was quite abysmal. The IOM published a follow up report (2004) emphasizing the need for safe care to be founded in the evidence of research, a term known in healthcare as "evidence-based practice." Updates in procedures, medications, and policy result from scientific research and peer review to validate "best practice." The IOM continues to advocate for patient safety and alert Americans of the state of unsafe medical practices that sadly continues today.

Although there have been many safety programs and new advanced technologies implemented by healthcare organizations in recent years, safety for patients remains elusive. Why do medical errors continue to occur at alarming rates? Despite these efforts at improving patient outcomes, the safety in our healthcare facilities has only minimally improved over the past several decades. There still remains a significant risk to you and your loved ones' lives in the healthcare system.

Medical Error Disclosure

Patient safety incidents or adverse events have occurred in nearly 42% of patients or their family members (O'Connor et al., 2010). In 2017, the IHI/NPSF found in a survey of 2500 people that 21%

of them have personally experienced medical errors; another 31% of Americans know someone who has been harmed by the healthcare system (https://www.ihi.org/about/news/Pages/New-Survey-Looks-at-Patient-Experiences-With-Medical-Error.aspx).

Moral and ethical guidelines are outlined in healthcare code of ethics principals and guide expected behaviors of medical personnel. "Autonomy and self-determination acknowledge the patient's right to make choices, to hold views, and to take actions based on personal values and beliefs" (Bonney, 2014). This ethical principle includes the patient's right to full information and to know if a medical error occurs. The principle of autonomy allows the patient to have full participation in their plan of care. Patients want an open and transparent conversation if an error occurs; they want and deserve an apology if a mistake was made. They need to hear from the physician what the plan of care is going forward after the mistake. Patients desire the information surrounding the medical error event; they want to know how and why it happened. They want to know the healthcare organization and the healthcare provider regret the mistake and that action will be taken to prevent further harm.

Physicians are obligated to disclose information about an adverse event to their patients. Frequently, they are reluctant or will avoid these conversations with patients or their families. Some healthcare providers believe that if the patient doesn't inquire about an event, they are not obligated to disclose (Ghazal et al., 2014). Unfortunately, healthcare providers are fearful to divulge details of the adverse event; this leads to many events going unreported. Litigation is a valid concern in many cases; doctors fear the very real, damaging impact to their reputation. Shame at making a mistake is a deep emotion felt by most healthcare providers in these situations; avoidance of the patient and the family is a natural reaction. Nurses fear punitive action will be taken when they report medical errors and do not trust needed changes will result from reporting (Africa & Shinners, 2020).

Physicians take the Hippocratic Oath, "first do no harm,"

at their white-coat ceremony signaling graduation from medical school. This oath is based on the ethical values of the medical profession to include confidentiality, beneficence, and non-maleficence. Shame makes us deceive. We want to avoid the patient and/or surviving family as much as possible, to get through our cleanup as quickly as possible, and get the hell away from it, to bury it, to forget about it" (Schlachter, 2017).

Studies have found that there are fewer lawsuits filed when doctors and hospitals offer an apology after a medical error occurs. "The desire for punitive measures is mitigated by the healthcare providers' approach in communicating an adverse event. An honest, empathetic, and accountable approach decreases the probability" of litigation (O'Connor et al., 2010). The University of Michigan Health System found a significant decrease in both medical malpractice claims and the cost of litigation when they implemented an open disclosure program (Kim & Lee, 2020).

Despite healthcare awareness and initiatives to move towards a "just culture" to support medical error reporting, little evidence exists that progress has been made towards this goal (Africa & Shinners, 2020). If the healthcare organization does not have a procedure of support in place for patient safety events, there is a great deal of uncertainty on how to manage the situation. Doctors are not infallible, but they have been socialized to believe that they should be. Ninety-eight percent of physicians agree that serious safety events should be disclosed; this doesn't seem to happen. Conversations about medical errors are not easy and can be very uncomfortable and challenging; most healthcare organizations do not have a clearly defined process to manage these events (Bonney, 2014).

Many physicians will give a partial account of the event, often misleading the patient and family away from the true nature of the adverse event. "There is a gap between ideal disclosure practice and reality" (O'Connor et al., 2010). Martinez et al. (2017) found that communicating a medical error or safety event to the patient and their family occurred "often" or "always" only in approximately 10%–30% of safety process leader meetings and conferences. What happens in the rest of these patient safety events? Are they just swept under the carpet in the hope that nobody finds out? I believe so; I've seen it happen.

Despite the implementation of safety programs in some healthcare facilities, it has been found that tools for analyzing adverse events have been underutilized. Martinez et al. (2017) submitted an analysis of "how clinical programs identified and reviewed adverse events and near misses" in a large academic medical center. Three categories of review panel approaches were identified: Morbidity and Mortality Conferences, Quality Assurance Meetings and Educational Conferences. An overall lack of disclosure and underreporting continues to persist in many healthcare facilities. There doesn't seem to be a structure of identifying adverse events, resulting in missed opportunity for quality improvement and future error prevention.

A deliberate and integrated safety culture is a *must* for health-care organizations and teams. Analysis of the root cause of the event is essential to identify medical errors and adverse events; as the saying goes, "An ounce of prevention is worth a pound of cure." A systematic approach is needed to review high alert occurrences (i.e., unplanned patient transfers to the intensive care unit, extended length of hospital stay, rapid response team calls, Code Blue calls). Organizations must identify system gaps and opportunities to provide further education and mentoring to identified individual healthcare professionals (Martinez et al., 2017).

Every single patient is someone's mother, father, daughter, or son, a member of humanity that deserves the utmost atten-tion and care. You should be empowered to be the advocate and gatekeeper of safety for your family and loved ones. Being armed with a little knowledge, fortitude, and courage to ask questions will help you be an advocate for safe care. The courage to speak up can literally be the difference between life and death. "The ability to learn from mistakes and make changes is an essential element of a safety culture" (Martinez et al., 2017).

Here are a few questions you may want to ask if you find yourself in this unfortunate circumstance. How are medical errors reviewed internally at the organization? What is the policy or law about disclosure? What should you expect from the healthcare team if a medical error occurs? Different U.S. states have different regulations; you'll need to research your state laws.

KEY TAKEAWAYS

- Safety is the freedom from accidental injury.
- Despite awareness and reporting of medical errors, very few changes have been made in how medicine is still practiced.
- 400,000 patients each year experience some level of preventable harm.
- The cost of medical errors is estimated at over $20 billion annually.
- 39% of adverse events are related to medication errors.
- 30% of adverse events are related to surgical procedures.
- *Never Events* (wrong site surgeries, etc.) should never occur but still cause devastation.
- Medical disclosure after patient harm frequently is only partially divulged (if at all).

CHAPTER 4

YOUR HEALTHCARE CONSUMER RIGHTS

What the Law States You Can Demand

In the 1970s, the American Hospital Association created the "Patient Bill of Rights" allowing patients to understand what they should expect when interacting with the healthcare system. This document was intended to empower patients and encourage their active participation in their own healthcare. Every patient has this basic set of rights to help them make decisions and ensure they are partnering in their plan of care. Understanding your rights as a patient is the first step to taking charge in directing and managing your health. Who is better than you in making these decisions than you?

In 1998, the U.S. Advisory Commission on Consumer Protection and Quality in Health Care Industry adopted the Patient Bill of Rights. It was deemed important that patients feel more comfortable in the U.S. health care system and it outlined three major pillars: 1) encourages patients to actively participate in their own health; 2) requires health care systems to meet patients' needs; and 3) provides an avenue for patients to address any concerns or issues they may have. Many health care facilities, insurance plans and even Medicare and Medicaid recognize the Patient Bill of Rights as expected standards of care.

The key areas of your Patient Rights are:

- The right to choose your healthcare providers (Chapter 5)
- The right to information that is easily understood and is accurate
- The right to respect and non-discrimination
- The right to be evaluated by emergency services if you feel your health is in danger
- The right to have your health information held confidential
- The right to have a timely and fair evaluation if you voice a complaint

Let's break down each of these areas and discuss in a little more detail.

Choosing your healthcare provider. Though there may be multiple providers you can choose to guide your healthcare journey, you may need to select a provider on your healthcare plan. You should find a provider that you feel comfortable with and one that you can trust; your doctor should have your health and best interest at heart. Ask the healthcare provider questions to determine if you feel listened to; you should feel you have been heard and understood. The doctor should collaborate with you in your health decisions. You need to feel safe and cared for, especially in potentially life-threatening situations.

Full Disclosure of Medical Error

When a medical error is realized, to "tell" or "not to tell" has been a moral and ethical discussion among healthcare professionals for decades if not longer. Fear of potential negative consequences and embarrassment influences the decision of some healthcare institutions and providers to conceal a mistake or harm to a patient. Healthcare ethical principles require a physician to disclose a medical error that may or may not cause harm to the patient (Ghazal et al., 2014). It is the patient's right to know if there has been a medical error during their care, whether harm was realized or not. Patients deserve disclosure and the knowledge to inform their decision-making; this is guided by the ethical patient right of self-determination and autonomy (Bonney, 2014).

Information that is easily understood and is accurate. Your right to information about your health includes everything from diagnostic test results, laboratory results, and potential or actual diagnosis. It is important that you create a plan of care in collaboration with your healthcare provider to maintain or restore your health. Your healthcare provider may utilize both simple and sophisticated assessments and diagnostic examinations to understand your level of health or illness. It's a bit like playing detective—the clues must be gathered and put together to create a picture of your health.

The terminology and words that physicians and nurses speak can seem like a foreign language to you. Sometimes healthcare providers may forget to translate this medical verbiage into "everyday" or layman's terms. If you do not understand a word, sentence, or concept, you *must* speak up and ask questions until you do comprehend what is being communicated to you. Do not feel intimidated or "stupid." Your healthcare providers have attended many years of schooling to learn their craft in the medical profession. Speak up and ask for clarification if you need to. The information that you receive about your health should be accurate and explained in a way that you can understand.

Respect and non-discrimination. Healthcare is a right of every human being; it is expected to be given to all equally without discrimination of race, religious beliefs, sexual preference or identity, gender, or age. Discrimination has been a hot topic in the media over the past few years; multiple examples of various types of discrimination have made headlines, stirred deep emotions, and incited many thoughtful conversations. Lawsuits citing discrimination have increased significantly in the past decade. In July 2022, a class action lawsuit was filed in Seattle, Washington, against a healthcare organization citing a consistent failure to ensure effective communication to deaf patients seeking medical care (https://dralegal.org/press/providence-health-filing/).

Unfortunately, discrimination in healthcare is more prevalent than previously determined. "Twenty-one percent of 2,137 American adults surveyed indicated they had experienced discrimination in the health care system; 72% of those who had experienced discrimination reported experiencing it more than once. Racial and ethnic discrimination was the most frequently reported type of discrimination respondents experienced" (Nong et al., 2020). At best, discrimination can lead to a barrier in receiving healthcare; at worst, it may contribute to a variety of deleterious or harmful outcomes.

Emergency evaluation and treatment. In the event you are experiencing a medical emergency, it is your right to receive an evaluation and treatment for your condition regardless of your financial status. The Emergency Medical Treatment and Active Labor Act (EMTALA) states that every patient entering the emergency department has the right to be seen and evaluated if they have an emergency. Additionally, EMTALA ensures that physicians cannot ask the patient for any proof of insurance or form of payment until after they are stabilized and treated.

As a healthcare consumer, you have the responsibility to take good care of your health with life choices and decisions you make each day. There are many resources available to help you find healthy food choices, smoking cessation methods, and simple exercise programs that can help you be your best physical self. You should also understand and follow the guidelines of your health plan to maximize the benefits that are yours as a health-care consumer.

There are also Bills of Rights for specialized areas, i.e., mental health and hospice. Some states in America have a specific Bill of Rights for their citizens. Here are general guidelines for your rights from the Medicare website:

Access to your personal health information. By law, you or your legal representative generally have the right to view and/or get copies of your personal health information from these groups:

- Health care providers who treat you and bill Medicare for your care
- Health plans that pay for your care, including Medicare

These types of personal health information include:

- Claims and billing records
- Information related to your enrollment in health plans, including Medicare
- Medical and case management records
- Other records that doctors or health plans use to make decisions about you

You should request a copy of your examination, and any diagnostic or laboratory results; it is your physician's responsibility to help you understand this information. You may have access to all your medical records; this is your personal information and it's yours upon request.

Timely and fair evaluation. Generally, you can get your information on paper or electronically. If your providers or healthcare plans store your information electronically, they must give you electronic copies if you ask for them. You have the right to get your information in a timely manner, but it may take up to 30 days to get a response. Keep in mind, if your information is electronic, you also have the right to have it sent to a third party of your choosing. A third party may be a:

- Health care provider who treats you
- Family member
- Researcher

You may have to fill out a form to request copies of your information and pay a fee. This fee can't be more than the total cost of:

- Labor for copying the information requested
- Supplies for creating the copy
- Postage (if you ask your health care provider to mail you a copy)

In most cases, you won't be charged for viewing, searching, downloading, or sending your information through an electronic portal (http://www.medicare.gov).

Take care of yourselves and your loved ones by understanding your patient rights. Become self-actualized by speaking up and taking charge of your personal medical health and the accompanying medical care you receive.

KEY TAKEAWAYS

- Understand your rights as a healthcare consumer—you have more than you know.
- Interview your potential healthcare provider to partner with you in your healthcare.
- Discrimination in healthcare occurs in up to 72% of patient encounters.

- Emergency Departments must render you care regardless of ability to pay.
- You have a right to access and understand your healthcare data.

CHAPTER 5

SELECTING YOUR HEALTHCARE PARTNERS

Doctors Aren't God and Hospitals Are Not Safe!

Brian J. has been a paramedic firefighter for over 23 years. He was working and had just brought a patient needing medical care to the hospital. Brian experienced a sudden onset of crushing chest pain (10/10) that radiated to his throat, diaphragm, and neck and was accompanied by sweating: a classic presentation for an Acute Myocardial Infarction (heart attack). A heart attack occurs when blood flow through the coronary arteries is impeded due to narrowing typically caused by a buildup of plaque on the inner walls of the artery. The plaque can break open in the coronary artery causing blood to clot in this area and preventing any blood from flowing through the artery.

Brian was assisted to the emergency department by his very concerned paramedic partner; he was admitted for evaluation. His initial electrocardiogram demonstrated abnormal findings of "possible" infarction and heart muscle injury. The reading from the ECG machine says "possible" because it cannot make a diagnosis; it is "smart" and indicates a cardiologist should be notified and is expected to examine the patient. The cardiologist "on call" was notified of Brian's admission, status, and results of the diagnostic exams (ECG, laboratory, and chest x-ray results). He did not come to the hospital to assess his patient with these reported critical findings.

Within less than an hour of admission to the Emergency Department, Brian's heart rhythm changed to atrial fibrillation with a rapid ventricular response at a rate over 120 beats per minute: a very unstable rhythm and concerning change! Brian's initial laboratory results indicated heart muscle injury; his troponin level was over 300 ng/m and kept climbing dangerously high with each subsequent lab draw. Troponin is considered the gold standard "heart attack" blood test, elevated troponin levels help practitioners to determine the severity of the heart attack. The normal reference range is listed as 0.00–0.40 ng/ml., 10 is considered a very positive indicator of a heart attack.

Brian's troponin levels were monitored very closely every few hours; they continued to escalate dramatically, indicating the damage occurring to his heart muscle. The cardiologist was given frequent updates on Brian's condition by the hospital staff; they alerted him to the critical changes occurring with this patient. The cardiologist *still* did not come to the hospital to assess and evaluate his patient with these critical findings.

Into the early evening, Brian's breathing became more labored; he was really struggling to breathe. His oxygen saturation had fallen dangerously low with readings in the 70s. His heart was so damaged due to lack of blood flow, it could not beat effectively. This is known as "pump failure" and resulted in fluid backing up into his lungs. He now had to be intubated to support his breathing; they inserted a breathing tube into his trachea, and he was placed on a ventilator. Brian's vital signs were deteriorating rapidly; he was started on multiple IV medications to sustain his blood pressure and keep him alive. He was transferred to the Intensive Care Unit for a higher level of care; his family watched over him, expecting him to die at any time.

Brian's wife sat at his bedside, horrified by the chaotic scene unfolding before her eyes; she saw him quit breathing and his blood pressure drop to 40/20! The cardiologist *still* did not come to evaluate and treat his critical patient. Just after 1:00 am, Brian's body gave out. He suffered a cardiac arrest, his heart stopped beating; he flatlined twice. Thankfully, resuscitation by the healthcare team was successful; Brian lived through the night.

The standard of care for an acute myocardial infarction is percutaneous coronary intervention (cardiac catheterization) for immediate diagnostics and intervention if indicated. If blockages in the artery are identified, an intervention using a balloon to open the artery and allow blood to flow through should be performed. Brian was at a hospital that boasts on their website: "Our hospital is accredited through The Joint Commission and the American Heart Association as a Primary Heart Attack Center." This means the hospital is dedicated to providing cardiac care with a patient-centric approach that is better for patients and their families. This hospital also lists the signs of a heart attack on their website—Brian exhibited exactly these symptoms when he arrived at their door. The Joint Commission describes the qualifications of a Primary Heart Attack Center as: "Recommended for organizations with on-site primary percutaneous coronary intervention (PPCI) coverage for patients 24 hours a day, 7 days a week."

When the cardiologist finally came to assess Brian at 7:00 am the following morning, they took him to the cardiac catheterization lab and found 2 of the 3 main coronary arteries occluded. Brian only had one coronary artery perfusing his heart with blood and oxygen. Because of the delay in the appropriate and the expected standard of care, Brian suffered heart failure and kidney failure; he is now blind in one eye due to a small blood clot in the artery of his eye. Why did it take the cardiologist *21 hours* to come and evaluate this critical patient?

In hindsight, Brian's wife states she wished she would have known she could escalate her fear that her husband was not getting the care he needed and could die. When the cardiologist refused to come to the hospital to treat her husband, she didn't know she could have asked to speak with the hospital House Supervisor. She could have escalated her desperation for someone to treat her husband's heart attack and demanded to speak with the Hospital Administrator on call. She felt powerless, helpless, and at the mercy of the system. Sadly, though Brian survived this catastrophic but preventable event, he will never work again in the profession he dearly loved—serving his community as a paramedic and a firefighter.

Choosing Your Physician

Physicians have a long history of presuming they know what is right for the patient; many patients have the belief that "the doctor knows best." The medical model and culture in America places doctors on a so-called pedestal. We have been socialized and taught to trust doctors; to "take them at their word." If you have blind trust and do not understand that all doctors are not equal, you may experience poor care and suffer undesirable health outcomes.

Some healthcare providers believe patients want the comfort of a doctor's authoritarianism; they believe that there is no valid reason for the patient to feel any uncertainty. This is a very dangerous attitude and can result in harm or may mean the difference between life and death. Your doctor should earn your trust; it shouldn't be given freely to the "title" of doctor. You must be a proactive patient and actively engaged in your own healthcare. You cannot afford to be naïve or assume anything when it comes to your health.

"Conversations that occur in doctors' offices or at a hospital bedside are some of the most critical any of us will ever have. The effectiveness of those discussions has a direct and measurable impact on individual patient health outcomes" (Awdish, 2018). As Dr. Awdish states in her book about her disastrous personal journey through the healthcare system, "We (doctors) weren't trained to listen. We were trained to ask questions that steered people to a destination. We were trained to value efficiency over cultivating a relationship through trust and disclosure. We weren't trained to value the patient's story."

Understanding this paradigm empowers you; knowing your rights as a patient and how to advocate for yourself and your needs is essential. Your doctor should take the time to listen to you; you should not feel rushed or feel confused about anything. You should feel comfortable with your physician; they should prioritize your health and safety as much as you do.

It is essential to select the right doctor to care for you and your family; you do have choices. All doctors make mistakes; they are human, but you can increase your safety by choosing your provider wisely. It is almost impossible to revoke a physician's medical license, so a doctor with a history of mistakes can take his license and relocate, most often to another state or small town. Medically underserved areas across the country can be so grateful to get a physician to provide healthcare to their community, they won't challenge his/her past or scrutinize his/her curriculum vitae too carefully. Patients can research their doctor's history and performance record; some states are now making it easier for you to find information on a physician.

Take the time to research a list of doctors, ask your friends for references, interview the candidate you want to entrust your health with. Ask questions about their experience with your health condition in particular; you want someone experienced with your health issue or disease. Getting to know your selected doctor is part of the vetting process; you need to see if they are the right provider to care for you.

If you know someone who works in a healthcare institution, they may have some "insider" information on certain physicians; ask their opinion about the physician's reputation. They will be careful though, as they will not want to jeopardize their own job.

When I worked in the Intensive Care Unit, there were doctors I decided I would never go to for my own medical care or refer a friend to. We as nurses see a variety of physician practices and attitudes; we found ourselves evaluating the doctors we worked closely with for care and competence.

Doctors may earn a negative reputation in healthcare circles if they demonstrate an uncaring or egotistical attitude towards patients. If they didn't listen to the patients or nurses, made questionable decisions (many would forego handwashing despite best practices and policy), or made mistakes without taking ownership, many colleagues did not trust them. We had a saying amongst the nurses for these types of doctors: "I wouldn't let him touch my dog." There were others who were reputable and really did care about their patients and had good outcomes; these were the ones from whom we would seek care and to whom we would refer our friends and family members.

There are benefits for choosing either a younger physician or a more seasoned and experienced physician. Medical knowledge was predicted to double every 73 days by 2020 (Denson, 2011); this has come true. Younger physicians that have a more recent education have likely learned about recently adopted innovative technologies and treatment modalities. However, younger physicians also do not have years of experience yet; keep that in mind. More mature and older physicians may have more experience treating a variety of patients, adding to a well-rounded experience. Unless they have regularly attended medical conferences and kept up on reading the current medical literature, older physicians may not be experienced in the newer technologies or options for treatments that are now available.

Regardless of the experience a physician may have, you want to look for doctors who treat you with respect and dignity. You want to feel that the physician listens to you. It is important they convey interest in you as a human being, as if your case is very important, because it is. Look for a physician who is honest and candid about his limitations. The doctor you choose should support their patients in being an active and full participant in their own health care and decision-making process.

A doctor who encourages your questions and explains things to your understanding is the partner you want in making decisions about your health. If you feel unsure about the recommendations your healthcare provider gives you, do some research and consult another provider. A good physician will not be upset or feel threatened by your questions or your desire to obtain a second opinion; they should encourage it when your health is at serious risk. You would be surprised how many different opinions there are for treating different medical conditions; you need to find the one that feels right for you.

Conversations with your doctor are some of the most critical you may have. Understanding how to effectively communicate with your physician will maximize the opportunity for you to receive the best healthcare. Here are a few guidelines to help facilitate your meeting with your doctor:

- Know your medical history.
- List your medications.
- Write down your questions, concerns, or issues before your appointment.
- State your fears if you are concerned about something— try to be direct.
- Make sure you understand what is explained and what is expected—restate for clarity.
- Continue to ask questions for clarification.
- Learn how to access your personal information and medical records on your patient portal.

Beware of any healthcare provider who displays any condescending attitudes or acts arrogant, won't let you ask questions or cuts you off in conversation, doesn't "listen," or treats you like you are "less than." These behaviors are unacceptable and can only cause you problems, or worse, may pose a threat to restoring your health. Egos can get in the way of communication if a physician feels he/she knows what's best for you without involving you in the discussion.

You want a doctor who is not too proud to ask questions when he doesn't know something; you want him to ask for help when he needs it. Medical knowledge doubles every few months and is quickly accelerating; doctors and nurses will never "know it all." These are the doctors who will make fewer mistakes; they don't let pride get in their way of caring for their patients. You want a doctor who feels a reverence for life; you want him caring for you as if you are family. Caveat emptor. Buyer beware.

If you are told you need to have surgery, you should be asking your surgeon specific questions. How many of these procedures have they performed in the past 12 months? Will there be any other surgeons or trainees in the operating room? If so, what exactly will be delegated to the lesser experienced of the two doctors (Schlachter, 2017)?

In healthcare institutions designated as teaching hospitals, there are interns and residents who are there to learn from senior doctors and surgeons. If you are having surgery, you want to be sure your surgeon is present and will have direct oversight and supervision over the resident physician. You would think this should be a reasonable expectation, but you would be surprised how often this doesn't actually happen.

As we previously discussed, wrong-site surgery occurs in U.S. hospitals approximately 40 times per week! The following information and patient guide can be found on the American College of Surgeons website to assist patients and their families (https://www.facs.org/for-patients/patient-resources/correct-site-surgery/).

Communication is the key. Discuss with your surgeon exactly what will be done before, during, and after your operation. Most of this information should be discussed with your physician before you sign the Informed Consent form, but do not hesitate to ask the following questions:

- What is the name of the operation that will be performed?
- Where or on what body part will you be operating?
- Are there any alternatives to this operation?
- What are the risks of this procedure?
- What is likely to happen if I don't have the operation?
- Who is in charge of the surgical team?
- About how long will it take to recover after the operation?
- What can I do to make sure the correct operation will be performed on the right place on my body?
- Will the correct part of my body be marked before the operation begins?

And don't stop there. Keep asking questions about anything you or your family want to know and until you fully understand everything that has been planned. Ask team members what role they will play in the surgery or procedure and in your care. Ask them what will they do to ensure your safety? You should carefully review your informed-consent form and verify the information on your patient identification bracelet.

Standards of Care

Despite the expectation most patients have of receiving restorative health care when they seek medical attention, this is not the always the experienced reality. Legally, the *standard of care* expects that a doctor only be *minimally competent.* "The law does not require that a doctor must be at least average, because if that were the case, half of all doctors would be in violation of the standard of care" (Schlachter, 2017). Shocking as it is, doctors and givers of medical care are not required to guarantee good results. Patients must be proactive and do their own thorough research and due diligence in selecting their health-care providers (Schlachter, 2017).

Because there are no codified "standards of care" against which juries can judge a doctor's performance, efforts have been made to tie it to clinical practice guidelines (CPGs). The preparation and dissemination of CPGs is a highly politicized process. The medical profession continues to model itself after ancient medieval guilds, where apprentices learned by observing the master of their craft.

Medical ethics and moral principles should guide professional behavior, care, and standards for healthcare providers. Beneficence is the expectation of "doing well" by giving competent care, the best care possible, and avoiding harm to patients (Ghazal et al., 2014). Today, there are guidelines for best practices in medicine, but they are not formal, written standards of care with reasonable expectations that you can find or obtain. When a physician is sued for malpractice, he has to convince the jury he met the lowest possible bar for quality care and should be exonerated. Really? Why would the lowest possible bar be an acceptable expectation for physicians? Would you take your beloved pet to a veterinarian that had a 1 out 5-star rating on a Yelp review?

In his book, *Malpractice: A Neurosurgeon Reveals How Our Healthcare System Puts Patients At Risk*, Dr. Schlachter (2017) describes a medical malpractice case where Abraham Lincoln was the attorney, defending a patient whose plaster cast was improperly applied. In this case, *Richie v West*, the Supreme Court of Illinois began to determine what patients should expect in healthcare: "When a person assumes the profession of physician and surgeon, he must . . . be held to employ a reasonable amount of skill and care."

Surgeons are a class of physicians that have extended their basic medical school education to include a surgical residency and a surgery fellowship. This specialty training gives them license to perform surgery; it does not guarantee that they are very experienced or are any good at it. For example, the research demonstrates that successful prostate surgery comes down to one thing: the experience and skill of the surgeon. Patients treated by highly experienced surgeons (defined as 250 or more surgeries performed) are much more likely to be cancer free five years after surgery (Potosky et al., 2004). "Twenty-five percent of all surgeons who perform this most delicate operation do only one per year, and 80% of all such surgeons perform 10 or fewer" (Schlachter, 2017).

Working in the healthcare environment can be extremely busy and stressful; unfortunately, shortcuts from "best practice" are adopted and practiced by nurses and physicians. Both nurses and doctors may routinely cut corners and don't see any harm in it. My nursing students have reported to me that the nurses in their clinical experiences have said, "I know what you were taught in school, but this is how we do it in the real world." This method of creating shortcuts and skipping steps may result in patient harm. The measure of a doctor's integrity is how high the stakes have to be before he stops telling the truth and starts lying (Schlachter, 2017). As we mentioned before, all and doctors and nurses make mistakes. And when they first start practicing, they make a lot of them.

Patients hope and expect that as doctors gain experience, they observe more, are able to identify different symptoms and types of diseases, and recognition patterns grow to arrive at the right diagnosis. Bias is seeing what you want to see or what you expect to see; this habit can cause a blind spot and may result in a physician missing a diagnosis or warning signs. Vigilance is essential for all levels of healthcare providers to prevent them from making mistakes and errors.

Google your doctor's name. Search for web sites that rate doctors and hospitals; read the reviews if you can find them. Ask your doctor about their professional experience; this can provide you with important insight. Ask about their background and where he/she has practiced medicine and where they have lived. You will know you have the right doctor when she/he welcomes your questions and shares information with you. You want a doctor who does not rush to reassure you and truly listens; you want them to share the basis for his/her clinical opinions. A good doctor will encourage you to get another opinion if you are hesitant at the suggested therapy or surgery.

Physician Fatigue

In the U.S., after completing medical school, graduates apply for "residency" to various specialty training programs around the country. Residency training programs give the newly graduated medical doctors the practical training and "hands-on" experience to bridge the theoretical knowledge learned in the classroom to practical application to patient care. Resident medical doctors typically work long hours and are frequently sleep deprived.

"Evidence shows that acute and chronically fatigued medical residents are more likely to make mistakes" (AHRQ, 2009). In 2011, a policy was enacted by the Accreditation Council for Graduate Medical Education (ACGME) restricting first-year residents from working over sixteen consecutive hours. Prior to this, many residents would work 24-hour shifts with another four hours for care transition (reporting to the oncoming provider).

In an environment requiring life and death decisions, a physician functioning for 28 hours without sleep is at significant risk of making mistakes that may lead to disaster. Degradation of performance in carrying out clinical tasks due to lack of sleep has been documented in the literature. With the implemented changes of mandatory work hours for first-year residents, Weaver et al. (2022) reported a significant decrease in harmful errors and patient deaths in a study of nearly 15,000 residents. The astounding improvements of patient outcomes when physicians received adequate sleep in this study demonstrated a 32% reduction of resident physician significant medical errors, a 34% reduced risk of preventable adverse events, and a 63% reduced risk of medical errors resulting in patient deaths.

Unfortunately, as of July 2017, ACGME lifted the work hours restrictions. The significant improvement of resident physician mental alertness and sharp cognition resulting in improved patient safety is again compromised. Mistakes and medical errors are bound to increase again, putting patient safety in jeopardy. The data suggests that resident physicians' exhaustion from long work hours contributed to 22,000 errors, 3100 of which led to preventable medical errors and 1500 patient deaths annually. It is recommended that medical residents should get ample sleep and adhere to 80-hour work week limits (AHRQ, 2009). Understanding the work hours expected of resident physicians and the potential for error, it is essential that you comprehend what role a medical resident will play in your or your family's healthcare. As they say, being forewarned is being forearmed.

Choosing a Hospital

Hospitals should be a safe place where patients can receive care that improves their health. All too often, the care patients receive can be sub-standard and even downright dangerous. In 2008, Medicare implemented changes to reimbursements to hospitals, including refusal to pay for a length of stay for patient care directly related to preventable complications. On the Hospital Compare website, the Centers for Medicare and Medicaid Services (CMS) provides consumers with publicly available information on the quality of Medicare-certified hospital care. The site includes specific information for both patients and hospitals on how to use the data to guide decision-making and improvement initiatives (https://www.medicare.gov/hospitalcompare/search.html):
Categories include:

- General Information
- Survey of patients' experiences
- Timely and effective care
- Complications and deaths
- Unplanned hospital visits
- Psychiatric unit services
- Payment and value of care

If you need to have surgery or need to undergo a procedure, choose a hospital or facility where many patients have had the procedure or surgery you need. Research shows that patients tend to have improved outcomes when they are treated in hospitals with more experience and those that are "specialized" in treating certain conditions (such as open-heart surgery, or robotic surgery). Depending on which health care facility the patient was admitted to, Your risk of dying depends on the hospital you choose. Based on the Leapfrog Hospital Safety Guide rating hospitals A–F, your risk of dying increases by 87.7% at a C grade hospital as compared to receiving care at an A grade hospital, and risk of death increases to 91.8% if you receive care at a D or F rated hospital (Austin & Derk 2019). (Leape, IHI, 2005).

The Leapfrog Hospital Safety Grades may inform patients on how a hospital prevents infections, what efforts are implemented to support healthcare teams, and identifies protocols and standards the hospital has put in place to prevent medical errors. They rate hospitals on the very basics of medical care and provide the following data for consumers:

- Frequency of personnel following handwashing guidelines
- Rate of hospital-acquired infections
- Utilizing computers to enter prescription orders (increases accuracy and decreases errors)
- Availability of highly trained nurses

KEY TAKEAWAYS

- If you have grave concerns about care being given or not given, escalate to the hospital House Supervisor and on-call Hospital Administrator if necessary.
- Research your physician; find one you can trust who respects your inquiries about your health.

- Get a second opinion if you have a serious health condition.
- Be prepared for your visit with your medical provider—bring your list of medications and past medical and surgical history.
- Ask detailed questions about your surgery—who will be present and what are their roles?
- Physician fatigue is very real—especially for resident or intern doctors. Sleep deprivation contributes to medical errors and patient harm.
- Research your hospital—know how they rate for safety and rates for infections.

CHAPTER 6

COMMUNICATION IS KEY

How to Have Crucial Conversations with Your Healthcare Team

Hand-off Communication

In 2013, Jennifer Nibarger suffered critical injuries in a boating accident; she was airlifted to a Level 1 Trauma Center to provide her with advanced care necessary to survive. Due to her extensive injuries, Jennifer needed a tracheostomy and a ventilator to assist her breathing. She experienced complications, setbacks, and challenges fighting a hospital acquired infection during her many weeks recovering in the hospital. Jennifer was able to finally make some progress in her recovery; she had finally turned the corner and was ready to be discharged home with the assistance of home health and rehabilitation. A "swallow test" was ordered to assess the trachea and airway because of the breathing tube she had in her throat for several months. The study showed she had a transesophageal fistula (TEF)—a hole between her trachea and esophagus allowing the passage of food or liquids into her lungs. This is a serious condition that requires surgery to close the hole and prevent life-threatening complications.

The barium utilized during the swallow study to identify the internal structure and tissue of the esophagus migrated through the hole in her trachea into her lungs. Jennifer experienced acute distress over the next several hours; her condition deteriorated as she struggled to breathe. Several times over the next few hours, she was transferred to various locations in the hospital. Jennifer continued to have respiratory difficulty and finally had to be placed back on the ventilator to help her breathe.

Unfortunately, the findings during the TEF were not communicated to the healthcare team. Jennifer's increasing shortness of breath was treated with anti-anxiety medications; the cause of her difficulty breathing was not identified until it was too late. The air and oxygen from the ventilator bypassed her lungs and went to her abdomen via the TEF. Jennifer now had experienced a lack of oxygen to her brain for over six hours, leading to permanent anoxic brain injury. Several weeks later, her family made the decision to discontinue life support. There was no hope for recovery from the medical error that occurred due to the devastating lack of hand-off communication.

The Joint Commission (2017) has cited communication failures among interdisciplinary team members as the most common root cause of sentinel events. "Handoff" communication is essential in healthcare practice to ensure vital information is passed between healthcare providers. "Walking rounds" have been adopted for shift change communication in many healthcare settings. This shift change procedure allows the off-going and on-coming nurses to walk from room to room together to see the patients and discuss pertinent events or needs the patient and family may have. This has been an effective strategy to augment the verbal report passed between nurses at shift change.

A common tool used in many healthcare facilities to improve the communication process is the SBAR (Situation, Background, Assessment, Recommendation); its purpose is to convey pertinent and concise patient information to improve continuity of care (Burke et al., 2020). Yes, it is important that the vital information is recorded in the patient's chart too, but verbal report is intended to discuss recent and pertinent information. Handoff communication should occur between nurses changing shifts, from ancillary departments to nurses, and between healthcare providers when there is relevant data that may impact the care and safety of the patient.

Healthcare Team Communication

Communication occurs when both the sender and receiver understand the message. Effective communication includes active listening, feedback, and is an engaging activity. There are many factors that may influence the effectiveness of the communication such as previous experiences, culture, emotional state, body language and tone. It is imperative for all healthcare providers and hospital staff to understand how effective communication contributes to patient safety; everyone from the CEO of the hospital to nurses, laboratory technicians, and respiratory therapists is responsible for patient safety.

Leaders in the healthcare industry have observed safety practices from other industries, most notably from the aviation industry. For many years, the culture of practice for airline pilots identified the chief or senior pilot as "pilot in command." He/she was in charge and made the decisions; the co-pilot did not question this authority. The co-pilot was expected to "follow orders," comply with the pilot's directives, and not to question a decision the pilot in command made. This culture began to change after a catastrophic event in 1977 in Tenerife, Canary Islands. KLM flight 747 crashed, killing all 583 passengers aboard, as told by John Nance in "Why Hospitals Should Fly."

In a coalescence of unfortunate events including fog, confusion and miscommunication surrounding this history-making event, the co-pilot was reluctant to speak up. The pilot heard from the tower that they were clear for takeoff; the copilot did not hear "clear" for takeoff from the tower. He had grave concerns in this disparity of the tower's message, he knew it could be a safety issue and impact the subsequent decision made by the pilot, but failed to assert himself. "The second officer never believed he had the permission, let alone the duty, to halt the captain and clear up the confusion" (Nance, 2008). In command of the aircraft was Jacob van Zanten, a senior pilot with thirty years of an untarnished aviation record. A long safety record can breed false assurance that a human being may be infallible when it comes to their area of expertise. John Nance calls this the Halo Effect—"the tendency to believe that someone more experienced and senior could not be wrong and you right."

In his book, John Nance reflects on this KLM flight tragedy and states, "the lack of communication, the misunderstood words, the pecking order obscuring vital information, and the assumptions not challenged—could have all occurred just as easily in any OR, ICU or any ER." Medicine is very hierarchical, especially in hospitals. Chief medical officers are at the top of the pyramid followed by department heads, senior attending physicians, lesser attending physicians, senior residents, followed by junior residents; at the bottom of this hierarchy are the interns and nurses. Each level of the healthcare team may feel fear when communicating with someone in a position of authority. Questioning a "superior" up the hierarchical chain has not been acceptable and certainly not encouraged in healthcare. Medical culture in general is still very hierarchical today in most healthcare settings; not questioning authority has been socialized and "taught" by example to be avoided at all costs. At times, that cost may be the life of a patient.

When I was a flight nurse on the trauma helicopter, I heard a saying that has forever stuck with me, "You can have an old pilot or you can have a bold pilot, but you will not have an old, bold pilot." This unfortunate fact came true in my experience when I was working in Las Vegas. We had a pilot with thousands of hours of flight experience; one night he chose to fly through a snowstorm, even when advised by his peers not to fly in the inclement weather. Flight crew "rules of the air" state that all crew members had to agree to fly or not to fly. I don't know why the flight nurse and flight medic on that fateful night agreed to leave the safety of the hospital and fly into a snowstorm.

That pilot crashed the helicopter not twenty minutes after launching off the hospital's helipad in an effort to return to home base; all three crew members perished that night. I've always wondered what the communication was between the three crew members. Did they trust the pilot's decision to fly into a snowstorm because of his years of experience and accident-free track record? I went to the crash site the following day; there were not even pieces big enough to hold in your hand from all the medical equipment on board or parts of the helicopter. It was just smashed into thousands of miniscule pieces. Such an unnecessary and preventable tragedy!

"The authority gradient can be a major hazard to patient safety" (Acquaviva et al., 2012). Nurses must feel empowered to speak up and find the courage to advocate for their patients. This is especially difficult when a physician dismisses the nurse's concerns when the situation is urgent, when the nurse knows or feels the patient's condition is in jeopardy or deteriorating. "Entrenchment in the medical hierarchy" has been reported as a significant barrier in healthcare team communication (Chua et al., 2020). Unfortunately, these situations are not isolated events and happen all too frequently.

Ineffective communication can negatively impact the patient's experience. It may result in increased length of stay for patients, increase adverse events, and decrease the level of satisfaction in patients, their families and those that provide health care (IHI, 2005). In one study, a change in mental status was documented in 37% of patients before cardiac arrest; the author noted "a common failure by the nurse to communicate the change to the doctor" (Schein et al., 1990). Nurses may fear being criticized or reporting information a physician may deem "unnecessary"; this may lead to a failure to communicate essential patient information to the physician in a timely manner (Chua et al., 2020).

A culture of "speaking up" between healthcare team members must be an organizational priority to promote a safe culture for patients. The fear of retaliation and feeling belittled silences many team members, whose concern should be voiced (Pattni et al., 2021). Despite the evidence found in the literature and as demonstrated in High Reliability Organizations, supporting the positive outcomes of an environment focused on equity of team members' contributions remains difficult in many organizations.

Advocacy

Patients place their trust in their physicians and healthcare providers; they believe hospitals are a safe place to receive care. The healthcare team has earned degrees and certificates in their specific area of expertise and has completed years of education and training in their respective fields. It is natural to place trust in physicians who have completed many hours of "hands-on training" as well as years of a didactic program to earn the educational degree. The traditional hierarchy in healthcare contributes to the discomfort of speaking up for many patients and family members; they have stated "It's not my place to question the team" (Bell et al., 2018).

Fear of the unknown is very real, and the healthcare environment is scary for many patients; many of these experiences fall into the "unknown" category. Many patients need support from family and friends to help make sense of this confusing world. Medical terminology is a special language that can sound very foreign; doctors and nurses sometimes forget to use understandable words and terms when conversing with patients. For example, "Your father's feet are very edematous today and that may be a symptom of CHF." Translated, this means "Your father's feet are very swollen with excess fluid today; it may mean his heart is not pumping adequately." Having a friend or advocate with them can help the patient remember or discuss what information was given to them about their treatment or diagnosis. Patients often feel overwhelmed and don't have control when they don't understand; "patient involvement is important patient safety practices" (Bishop & Macdonald, 2017; Harris et al., 2020).

Bell et al. (2018), report that 50% to 70% of patient families surveyed in the ICU setting reported feeling uncomfortable or afraid to voice their concerns about their loved one's care. Patients who are ill are a very vulnerable population; they are reliant on the healthcare team to care for them so may be reluctant to speak up and question the healthcare staff and physicians. Patients may believe if they are the "good patient," they will receive better care (Sutton et al., 2023).

Involving patients in their own healthcare plan creates an environment of inclusion and teamwork; it provides an opportunity for continuity of care, collaborative conversations, and accuracy of pertinent data. Improved patient outcomes occur more frequently when patients and their families are involved in decisions and delivery of healthcare. Patients reported feeling as if they were "objects of treatment" when uninformed of the plan of care (Bishop & Macdonald, 2017).

Family members report "not knowing how to raise my concern or who to talk to" (Bell et al., 2018). Critically ill patients may not have the capacity to advocate for themselves or ask appropriate questions. Your loved ones may need you to help them express their concerns, their needs, and to formulate questions for the healthcare team, especially when something doesn't feel "right." Don't second guess yourself when something feels "off," or you just need more information.

Many patients know their bodies and how "normal" feels to them, especially if they live with a chronic medical condition. They may "feel" when something isn't quite right; physicians and nurses should partner with patients and respect the individual and their experience. The consequences of not "speaking up" when you feel or know something is wrong or not quite right can have devastating consequences. The healthcare team really does need your help!

David was a patient admitted to the Emergency Department with chest complaints; the chest symptoms improved, but his breathing was getting worse. His physicians disregarded the patient's concerns and requests to check him for heart failure; he knew what the swelling in his legs and feet meant in the past. Finally, an echocardiogram was ordered and revealed David did in fact have heart failure and a critically low function of his heart muscle. David was subsequently given the appropriate care and treated with medications to improve his condition; this should have been a more collaborative conversation resulting in an improved outcome much sooner (Sutton et al., 2023).

Families are often ones that recognize early or subtle changes in the patient's condition. They typically are familiar with the nuances of their family members and may identify key clues the healthcare team may not notice. Safety issues are crucial to report; timeliness is essential to ensure the best outcome for the patient. Ideally, families will partner with the healthcare team in providing essential and individualized information about the patient, thus supporting them to improve patient care (Bell et al., 2018).

Ask Questions

As discussed in Chapter 4, it is your right as a patient to have information about your health and your body given to you in a way that you can understand. It is also your right to make decisions that will affect your health and your body. To make good decisions that are right for you, you must be able to understand the language of your healthcare provider and its implications for you. Patients and families perceive the authority gradient or medical hierarchy when conversing with physicians; many have been afraid to ask questions or to ask for clarification.

Frequently, the healthcare providers spend only a few minutes with the patient and seem to be always in a big hurry. Don't let this behavior deter you from understanding their plan to restore you back to health.

Be assertive but respectful when asking for information from your healthcare providers. Position yourself as partnering with them to work together for the best outcome for yourself or your loved one. This is not about challenging their competency as a healthcare provider; it's about partnership and teamwork! An example of what you might say to the physician could be "I noticed that my dad is having more trouble breathing this morning, what do you think?" The physician or nurse should answer you and share the patient's assessment and relevant data, for example, "The chest x-ray looked a little better this morning and the lab work is improving." If you still feel uncomfortable, ask "What do his lungs sound like? Does it sound like he has fluid in his lungs?"

Here is a link of short videos to show you how some patients and their families asked simple questions to help them get the right care they needed and improve their experience with the healthcare team: https://www.ahrq.gov/patients-consumers/patient-involvement/ask-your-doctor/videos/index.html.

Provide Information

Make sure that all your healthcare providers have your important health information; this includes any allergies you may have, all your medications, past surgical history, and medical history. Do not assume that everyone has all the information they need as most systems housing medical records do not share data. There are many "apps" for your phone that you can use to enter all your pertinent health information; it can be difficult to remember all your medications or dates of your surgeries.

Your healthcare provider should be discussing your healthcare plan with you and the prescribed goals of the therapy. The conversation should include the medications that have been prescribed for you and the intended effects. You should understand the purpose of the diagnostic and laboratory examinations your doctor has ordered that will be performed. You should understand when to expect the results of all diagnostic and laboratory tests; you should also expect to understand the meaning of the results and the significance to your health. Your healthcare provider should tell you the expected outcomes of the treatments ordered and the expected length of stay in the hospital. It will be important to take notes; I recommend bringing a loved one or friend with you to help you remember what was discussed.

Speaking up is a vital component of communication in the healthcare setting. You know yourself or your family member better than anyone; you may be the first to know that something is wrong or "not normal." If you *feel* (yes, intuition is very real), that there is something wrong or you feel worried or alarmed about something, it is imperative that you tell everyone caring for you or your loved one. The importance of integrating patients and their families into the healthcare culture of safety is growing in awareness and is being implemented in many healthcare facilities.

The Joint Commission has developed programs for the healthcare consumer which can be found at: https://www.joint-commission.org/topics/speakup_about_your_care.aspx.

If your family member's condition is changing or is "not right" and you feel concerned it is not being addressed or taken seriously, you have the right to request an evaluation from the Rapid Response Team (discussed in Chapter 8). This team is trained and equipped to respond very quickly in the event of an urgent situation or real emergency. Many facilities have the phone number posted for families to call in the event they believe there is a grave concern about the patient's condition. When you or a loved one are admitted to the hospital, ask the question: "What is the number I can call if I feel my family member or loved one is in acute distress?" I hope you never need it, but it is best to be prepared.

Escalation of Concern

Helen Haskell, Lewis Blackman's mother, in our opening story, knew something was wrong with her son. She did not know who to escalate her concerns to about Lewis's condition; she had already shared her concerns and anxiety with Lewis's nurses and resident physician, but effective action was not taken. They were the ones caring for Lewis at his bedside; it was a logical conclusion for her to believe that this was enough, and they would attend to her son's condition. Helen Haskell didn't know that nurses had a supervisor that she could ask to speak to when Lewis's condition deteriorated. She didn't know that doctors would have a phone number she could call with her concerns (as they were hospital doctors).

Who do you talk to if you are not getting answers to your questions or resolutions to your problems? There is a hierarchy in medical care and there is always someone else you can call or ask to speak to. If you do not get answers from your healthcare provider, keep asking until you do get the answers. Nurses have a charge nurse and a unit manager. Hospitals have a nurse designated as "House Supervisor" to ensure smooth operations and proper patient care. Resident physicians have chief residents to consult with. If you need to (as in Lewis Blackman's case), insist the chief resident call the primary or attending physician or the surgeon. There is always a hospital administrator "on call"; insist this person be notified if you are having an emergency.

Speak up! Do not be afraid to, and when you ask questions, make sure you understand the answers, and take a stand for the health of yourself and your loved ones. If your intuition or your gut instinct is telling you something isn't right, take your concern to the next level and the next level after that. Don't give up until your question is answered or your situation is resolved. And don't let the system intimidate you; your loved one's life may be in danger.

KEY TAKEAWAYS

- Hand-off communication between healthcare providers and ancillary departments is essential.
- Authority gradient—do not be afraid to question the physician. Harm may occur to you or your loved ones if you do not speak up.
- 50 to 70% of patient families reported feeling uncomfortable or afraid to voice their concerns about their loved one's care. Speak up!
- Be assertive, respectful, and professional in conversations with the healthcare team.
- Be an advocate—listen and provide support for your family member. Don't give up.
- Escalate your concerns if you need to—when something doesn't feel right, get answers, and insist on action.

CHAPTER 7

FAILURE TO RESCUE

Why Don't They Notice When You Start to Die?

A 67-year-old patient was admitted for surgery to repair non-healing fractures in both of her heel bones after falling off a ladder six months prior. The surgery went well; the patient did need several pain medications to manage her pain as she had built up tolerance to the pain medications over the six months after the accident. She became quite anxious during physical therapy and was prescribed Ativan (lorazepam). On the second day after surgery, she was confused and making inappropriate comments, had trouble breathing, and complained her leg pain was "10/10." The patient continued with very restless behavior, taking off her oxygen mask even when the nurse reapplied it, explaining the oxygen was needed; the patient stated "I just can't sit still." The patient's family was very concerned and asked the physician to come and evaluate her. She was taken to the radiology department for a chest X-ray due to the sound of fluid in her lungs and arterial blood gases indicating a lack of oxygen in her blood.

The patient's respiratory rate was now 48 breaths per minute; she was given a low dose diuretic medication to get rid of extra fluid and ease her breathing. The respiratory therapist charted a respiratory rate of 32 breaths per minute after a breathing treatment was administered. There was no communication of concern to the physician; there was no follow-up action, or any close observation initiated. Yes, a respiratory rate of 32 is an improvement over a rate of 48 but is still critical! The physician ordered labs to be drawn but the results were not checked; her low potassium levels were not noted or treated. The diuretic medication she was given (Lasix) causes potassium to be excreted and will further decrease potassium levels. Potassium is critical for normal cardiac function and must be replaced when levels are below normal. Her chest X-ray results showed congestive heart failure; these concerning results were not observed or noted by the physician or the nurse. The patient's rapid breathing continued for over three hours; the respiratory fatigue resulted in respiratory failure. She was found dead a short time later (Zimmerman, 2008).

The brain is the most sensitive organ of the body; when it does not receive enough oxygen, the patient may get restless, anxious, and confused. Any confusion or mental status change lasting longer than ten minutes may indicate that immediate action should be taken to explore the cause (Zimmerman, 2008). Many opportunities to intervene in this patient's deterioration were missed. Sadly, this patient's death was avoidable and could have been prevented hours before she died.

"Patient deterioration can be defined as an evolving, predictable and symptomatic process of worsening physiology towards critical illness" (Lavoie et al., 2014). Patient deterioration is *solely* a physiological phenomenon; this means there is *observable* evidence of clinical instability indicating interventions must be implemented rapidly (Lavoie et al., 2014). *All* patients have the potential to become critically ill; observance and monitoring is vital in all aspects of patient care.

Failure to Rescue (FTR) is the unexpected death of a patient that could have been prevented (Verillo & Winters, 2018). FTR is a phenomenon defined in the literature as failure to prevent the death of a patient by *failing to recognize, communicate or act on signs of physiological deterioration* resulting from an underlying illness or surgery (Jones et al., 2011; Lavoie et al., 2014; Levett-Jones et al., 2010). At the fundamental level, FTR equates to a failure of implementing the appropriate action to stabilize the declining patient (Garvey, 2015).

Physiological deterioration occurs over the course of several hours or longer; it follows a predictable path of symptoms that are amenable to intervention if detected early enough. Decades of research indicate that *observable evidence* of clinical instability and patient deterioration frequently occurs from 6–24 hours prior to cardiac arrest (Hodgetts et al., 2002; Simmonds, 2005; Thielen, 2014; Fasolino & Verdin, 2015; Mushta et al., 2018). Panday et al. (2017) found abnormal vital signs have frequently been documented up to 24 hours prior to a cardiac arrest event. Hodgetts et al. (2002) cited there was observable deterioration eight hours before cardiac arrest in up to 84% of the cases reported. In 99 out of 150 cardiac arrest cases in Alabama and Florida institutions, the patients showed signs of deterioration during the six-hour period before the cardiac arrest occurred (Farhat, 2008). Contrary to popular belief, sudden cardiac death is not very common.

In 2007, FTR was recognized as a patient safety indicator (PSI) by the Agency for Healthcare Quality and Research, urging healthcare organizations to recognize and prioritize this quality care metric. Critical assessment of patients prior to deterioration requires critically thinking nurses and healthcare providers, not merely the act of gathering and recording of vital signs (Roney et al., 2015). Insufficient patient surveillance, situational awareness, and vigilance has been linked to increased FTR, patient complications, and death (Herron, 2017; Labrague et al., 2022). Unfortunately, patients continue to die a preventable death due to lack of significant interventions and safety programs implemented by healthcare systems in the past several decades.

More attention and focus are needed to detect patients who are declining to avert impending crisis (Mushta et al., 2018). When the patient begins to physiologically deteriorate and there is no response or action taken by the nurse or healthcare provider, respiratory arrest and cardiac arrest may ultimately occur. Suboptimal care is ascribed to a failure to monitor the patient's basic clinical and physiological parameters. Failure to detect changes in a patient's condition is an ongoing patient safety concern across the continuum of care; it is fraught with potential harm to patients and even death if the deterioration goes unnoticed.

FTR Is Comprised of Three Components

- Failure to Recognize
- Failure to Act
- Failure to Communicate

FAILURE TO RECOGNIZE

To "rescue" a patient from deterioration, the nurse must be alert to early changes in the patient's vital signs, neurological status, and other important assessment data. "If all nurses were to adapt the primary survey approach (assessment of airway, breathing, circulation, and disability as the first element of patient assessment), they would be more focused on active detection of clinical deterioration rather than passive collection of patient data" (Considine & Currey, 2015). A focused assessment utilized by the healthcare team together with timely collaboration and communication during the "golden hours" of patient deterioration is crucial to saving lives (Ghaferi, 2017).

The correlation in observed physiological changes and patient cues is highly dependent on the nurses' ability to critically think and understand the implications of the data (Kyriacos et al., 2011). Mok et al. (2015) found that 25% of nurses thought that the patient's blood pressure was the most significant indicator of impending patient deterioration, but research has established the patient's respiratory rate is the most significant indicator of patient instability (Garvey, 2015). Caring for patients requires surveillance—purposeful and ongoing acquisition, interpretation, and synthesis of data for clinical decision making (Shever, 2011). When surveillance and nursing observations of patients occur twelve or more times as compared to less than twelve times a day, it results in a significant decrease in cases of FTR and thus greatly improves patient outcomes (Burke et al., 2022).

Subtle changes in a patient's level of awareness or orientation may indicate a patient is becoming unstable; it should alert the nurse to gather more data and investigate further. A new state of confusion is a blatant sign the patient needs immediate intervention (Garvey, 2015). If a patient asks, "What time is it?" for the third time in ten minutes, and this is a change for this patient, further evaluation is necessary. There may be various causes leading to changes in a patient's mental status; low levels of oxygen or low blood sugar levels can manifest as confusion or restlessness. More serious events such as bleeding in the brain may cause a patient to become confused, disoriented, or even unconscious. Any concerning changes or unusual observations should be investigated or reported to the physician.

Vigilance is the art of "watching out"; it is the attention to and identification of clinically significant observations, signals and clues collected from the patient's physiological data. This watchfulness should be part of every nurse's thinking process while they are completing the necessary tasks in caring for patients (Meyer et al., 2007). The nurses should be thinking, "What might happen to the patient if I don't address this concern?" For example, if a chest tube drainage container has a higher-than-expected amount of drainage or a change in color of the drainage, the nurse should notice this as a potential problem and must take action.

To understand the patient's physiological condition, the nurse needs to know what relevant patient information and data to collect and must be able to derive meaning from the collected data. It is essential the nurse understands the pertinent or priority data; this data needs to be analyzed with a critical thought process. For example, if the patient has an increased heart rate, the nurse needs to utilize critical thinking to determine the meaning of the data. Is the patient dehydrated or experiencing pain? Is the patient's blood pressure low and causing the body to compensate, resulting in an increased heart rate? The healthcare provider needs to determine what may be causing the abnormal physiological data and intervene as necessary. When data is collected and entered in the patient's chart, it must be compared and analyzed to determine if it is normal for this patient or a cause for concern. Is it expected or unexpected? Is it chronic or acute? Is the patient symptomatic?

FAILURE TO ACT

A basic understanding of pathophysiology, the physiology of abnormal states, is foundational knowledge taught in the very beginning of nursing school. Comprehension of normal body functions and the changes that occur in response to a disruption of homeostasis, is the foundation of recognizing early risk of patient harm. Understanding the body's response to a change is a prerequisite for deciphering the observed physiological cues when a patient begins to deteriorate. Timely and appropriate action is necessary by the nurse, doctor, and the healthcare team to significantly impact patient outcomes (Burke et al., 2022).

Recording vital signs and physiological patient observations is not enough if abnormalities are detected (Dalton et al., 2018). The nurse must take immediate and deliberate action to mitigate the decline of the patient's condition. Studies show that nurses and doctors do not have sufficient understanding of recognition of the impact of monitoring patients' vital signs in caring for patients. "Monitored vital signs with trend analysis could improve the prediction of deterioration prior to a serious adverse event" (Brekke et al., 2019).

Meaningful action can vary depending on the patient's condition. If the patient is short of breath, the head of the bed should be elevated to assist breathing (if not contraindicated). If the patient is in distress, the next action the nurse should take is collecting more patient data to determine the urgency of the situation. For example, if the patient's respiratory rate is noted to be elevated or rapid, what is the patient's heart rate? What do the lungs sound like when listened to with a stethoscope? What is the oxygen saturation level? What is the patient's level of consciousness? Absence of intervention to address physiological changes may lead to a patient's harm and potential death.

If the nurse or healthcare provider does not utilize critical thinking to synergize the data or assess the patient further, they may not "notice" the patient's physiological deterioration. The goal is to observe and be alert to the earliest shift in the patient's condition; this is the time when interventions can positively impact the patient's outcome. Early assessment and early intervention save lives.

Asking for help from the healthcare team may be necessary when the patient begins to deteriorate and becomes unstable. Taking focused action with the healthcare team to communicate and organize the immediate care of the patient is paramount for the patient to experience a good outcome. Resources must be mobilized to intervene, correct or reverse the patient deterioration (Ashcraft, 2004). It takes a cohesive and collaborative healthcare team to help the patient through the distressing situation. In the next chapter we will discuss Rapid Response Teams designed for this very purpose of supporting the healthcare team in these situations.

FAILURE TO COMMUNICATE

Failure to notify the physician and/or being unsuccessful in communicating the seriousness of the situation can lead to the patient dying. Ineffective communication can result in increased length of stay for patients, increase adverse events, and decrease the level of satisfaction in patients, their families and those that provide health care (IHI, 2005). When the patient's condition is becoming unstable, communicating with **CUS** words are a tool to convey urgency and get the healthcare team's attention: I'm **Concerned** about, I'm **Uncomfortable** because . . . , this is a **Safety** issue. Outlined in each state's Nurse Practice Act, the nurse is responsible to be the patient's advocate. If the patient's physician does not respond in a timely manner to a nurse's concern about a patient's status, it is expected and is a nursing standard of care for the nurse to escalate concerns up the medical chain of command.

Documentation in the patient's chart of communication attempts is necessary but the nurse cannot stop there. If the patient condition is unstable, the nurse must persist in advocating for the patient until help arrives (Zimmerman, 2008). Research indicates that when nurses communicate urgent information with a physician, it is most effective when the message is delivered in a confident manner and when "medical language" or terminology is utilized. It is vital to get the physician's attention when a patient is unstable; packaging the pertinent data in a succinct and clear manner should facilitate desired action (Andrews & Waterman, 2005).

TeamSTEPPS (Team Strategies and Tools to Enhance Performance and Patient Safety) is a program many hospitals utilize to teach and promote techniques for team communication to improve patient safety. These guidelines state that a nurse must assertively voice a concern at least twice, taking stronger action if the patient's problem remains unresolved. I recommend this method for family members too; don't stop until you feel you've been heard, and the healthcare team is taking action.

FTR rates increase in hospitals with higher nurse-patient ratios; these staffing shortages present a difficulty and even indicate an inability to closely monitor patients. When staffing ratios are inadequate to care for the complexity of the patient on the ward, adverse events are more likely to occur. Higher incidence of cardiac arrests happens on medical-surgical units; 35–40% of unexpected deaths occur on the medical/surgical unit (Rutherford et al., 2004). The nurse/patient ratio and the lack of experience of nurses working in the medical/surgical wards likely contribute to the incidence of unexpected deaths in these areas. Early detection of changes in vital signs and neurological status with appropriate intervention can help avert subsequent cardiac arrest (Genardi et al., 2008). Clinical signs of deterioration were considered to have been acted upon partially in 53% of cases, and not acted upon in 48% of the cases of cardiac arrest (Hodgetts et al., 2002).

The acuity of patients that are cared for on the medical/ surgical wards has increased over the past several decades (Wood, 2019). Patients are being transferred from the ICU to the medical/surgical areas earlier in their recovery than in past years; these patients are at higher risk for adverse events (Kyriacos et al., 2011). Patients admitted from the Emergency Department to general care floors are "sicker" than ever before. The staffing ratio of patients to nurses is a concerning factor on the medical/ surgical units; more patients are assigned to an individual nurse in these areas, putting them at increased risk of unrecognized deterioration. Sixty-eight percent of all FTR deaths occur among surgical inpatients with treatable complications such as pressure ulcers, post-operative respiratory failure, and post-operative sepsis (Reed & May, 2011).

Failure to detect changes in a patient's condition is an ongoing patient safety concern across the continuum of care (ECRI, 2019). Many nurses caring for patients on the general care floors are inexperienced and under-skilled; they have heavy workloads and are many times hampered by caution. When these nurses are unsure of "what to do," frequently they don't do anything.

In exploring processes contributing to failure to rescue in hospitals, Hughes (2004) cites cases where there were nurses who knew with complete certainty that immediate action was needed but didn't take action. These nurses state they felt constrained by policies and regulations preventing them from acting to help the patient without physician authorization. Cioffi (2000) reports that many nurses surveyed after FTR events occurred stated they felt uncertain about calling the physician or supervisor for help; they were worried about "doing the right thing" or "looking stupid" to their peers and medical team.

Hodgetts (2002) reported approximately 80% of patients who suffer a preventable cardiac arrest in the hospital do not survive. Cooper et al. (2012, 2013) stated that 80% of cardiac arrests are preventable. Mok et al. (2015) found 84% of cardiac arrests were potentially avoidable. In another study, a change in mental status prior to the event was found in 37% of arrest patients; the author notes "a common failure by the nurse to communicate the change to the doctor" (Schein et al., 1990).

The literature reveals that nurses may have little confidence in their ability to accurately assess a deteriorating patient; they may take the "wait and see" approach before calling the physician with their concerns. Even nurses with years of clinical experience may not report patient deterioration in a timely manner. Hart et al. (2014) found only half of the nurses with an average of 13 years of clinical experience felt confident in their ability to recognize the signs of patient deterioration.

There may be a delay in appropriate care and intervention when nurses report abnormal clinical observations to resident or junior doctors rather than senior providers (Kyriacos et al., 2011). Many nurses believe that a physician (even a junior or novice physician) is the "authority," and may not speak up or question them about decisions or orders received (Dalton et al., 2018). Effective communication may be impacted by feeling uncomfortable or afraid to voice concerns to someone perceived to be higher up on the medical hierarchy. Unfortunately, this is not uncommon when the nurse is inexperienced or lacks clinical skills and knowledge to manage the care of a deteriorating patient (Allen, 2020).

Clinical Reasoning

Good patient outcomes are directly related to the nurse's ability to recognize early signs of patient deterioration. Acting on the patient assessment, patient data collected and effectively communicating the urgency of the patient's condition to the physician or healthcare provider is paramount in saving lives. Clinical reasoning is an essential component in preventing FTR and should be emphasized in nursing education and new graduate orientation.

Clinical reasoning is the ability of nurses to consider and make sense of assessments and patient trends, combined with previous patient experiences to recognize significant changes in a patient's clinical condition (Herron, 2017). Action must accompany the recognition of a decline in the patient's condition. Application of appropriate nursing interventions is imperative in the patient safety process.

The nurse must utilize the knowledge learned in school and gained with clinical experience to anticipate what complications are likely to occur. For example, a patient with the diagnosis of heart failure from a weakened heart muscle is prone to fluid overload. In this condition, because the heart can't pump all of the blood out to the body, some fluid may back up into the lungs, causing difficulty breathing. Caution must be taken when intravenous fluids are administered, even when medically indicated; the extra fluid may jeopardize the patient's ability to breathe and oxygenate adequately. Rescuing a deteriorating patient is only effective if nurses have the knowledge and the skills to understand the urgent actions necessary for intervention (Hart et al., 2016).

I was working with students in the hospital setting several years ago, helping the students apply the classroom learning to the clinical environment. The clinical experience exposes and immerses the students in applying their acquired knowledge to the process of caring for patients. One of the patients we were caring for had a medical history of congestive heart failure and was receiving a blood transfusion. During the infusion of the first unit of blood, the patient's respiratory rate started increasing and she began having some difficulty breathing. Understanding the infusion of any fluid (including blood) could potentially place a burden on a patient's weakened heart muscle. We listened to her lung sounds and heard crackles, a sure sign of extra fluid in the lungs.

If the heart can't pump effectively because it is weakened or enlarged, the excess fluid may backflow into the patient's lungs. We placed a call to the physician and received an order to give Furosemide, a medication to increase urine production, resulting in an easing of the workload on the heart. The patient's kidneys responded quickly and started producing more urine; we were grateful that she began breathing easier and became more relaxed. Had we not been vigilant, anticipating a potential complication and paying close attention, this could have resulted in a real emergency for this patient.

Clinical Judgment

Clinical judgement is developed as the nurse accumulates experience, gains knowledge, and utilizes skills in caring for patients; this leads to the nurses' ability to synthesize patient data for appropriate clinical decision-making. It is frequently utilized during a nurse's daily tasks in caring for patients. Recently, nurse educators have revised nursing curriculum and integrated a clinical judgment model into the classroom and clinical settings. Students need to be prepared to care for the population of patients they will encounter in the healthcare setting; the acuity of patients demands well-trained nurses to improve patient outcomes and save lives.

In essence, Failure to Rescue is a direct result of the nurse's inability to utilize clinical judgment. As the nurse is the patient's primary care giver and spends the most time at the patient's bedside, the responsibility for recognizing patient deterioration and preventing FTR fall directly on nurses' shoulders. Unfortunately, FTR is not part of nursing education, nor is it a part of medical school curriculum. Perhaps we will see the cases of FTR decrease when nurses utilize the principles of clinical judgment, critical thinking, and clinical reasoning in caring for every patient.

It has been recommended by numerous researchers and healthcare advocates that training healthcare personnel to recognize the deteriorating patient must be a part of mandatory annual training for nurses and should be a part of health policy reform (Waldie et al., 2016). There would be an enormous opportunity and overarching benefit for all patients if this concept were adopted in all health sciences educational programs.

The Agency for Healthcare Research and Quality (AHRQ) has developed Patient Safety Initiatives to identify factors found to contribute to medical errors:

- Failing to follow policies and procedures in caring for patients
- Failing to properly identify patients when giving medications
- Failure in performing treatments or performing inaccurately
- Failure to complete patient assessments (Van Den Bos et al., 2015)

Lewis Blackman's case at the beginning of this book is an example of failing to adequately assess a patient on multiple occasions. If the nurse and resident physicians would have performed a proper assessment, they would have noted his distended and firm abdomen (clearly not a normal finding), his abnormal vital signs indicating he was in shock, and Lewis's complaints of abdominal pain that continued despite receiving pain medications. There were multiple *missed opportunities* to save Lewis's life.

Post-surgical patients are at extremely high risk for FTR; Dr. Silber in 1992 recognized and subsequently studied this phenomenon. Healthgrades noted in a 2013 report that 10% of Medicare patients undergoing surgery are at risk of dying from pulmonary embolus (blood clots that travel to the lungs), pneumonia, sepsis (blood infection), shock that may lead to cardiac arrest, and gastrointestinal bleeding.

Most of the FTR cases occur within 48 hours of arriving at the medical surgical unit (Verrillo & Winters, 2018). All of these complications can be identified by observing and acting on the early signs of patient deterioration. Early detection of physiological deterioration decreases patient length of stay, improves outcomes, avoids potential litigation, and saves lives.

Patient safety organizations such as the National Quality Forum, the Joint Commission, and the Agency for Healthcare Research and Quality have highlighted the frequency and threat of respiratory failure after surgery. Postoperatively, a combination of the effects of anesthesia and medications for pain control may contribute to these patients being at risk for poor outcomes. National standard guidelines have been created by patient safety organizations and disseminated to healthcare agencies highlighting these risks; massive and rapid change is required to diminish and eliminate unnecessary patient deaths.

Key Physiological Parameters to Monitor

- Vital Signs
- Oxygen Saturation
- Level of Consciousness
- Fluid Balance (urine output, intravenous fluids)
- Critical lab values
- New, unexpected, or unusual pain
- Altered skin color and/or skin temperature

Each of these key parameters will be discussed in further detail in subsequent chapters. These essential elements of patient assessment are vital to capture the early signs of deterioration that many healthcare providers miss. Abnormal physiological observations are "the most important manifestation of existing or developing critical illness" (Ryan et al., 2004). If the nurse and healthcare team do not recognize the urgency of the situation, the patient may continue to deteriorate and require resuscitation. Often, by the time the patient is exhibiting late signs of deterioration, it may be too late to reverse and cardiac arrest may ensue.

Vital sign measurements, tracking, and trending are critical to identify early signs of patient instability. For example, tachycardia, a heart rate above 90 beats per minute, may be a result of dehydration or excessive bleeding, or may indicate an early onset of shock. An increasing respiratory rate of over 20 breaths per minute requires vigilance; a trend of increasing respiratory rate of 24 breaths per minute and higher may be an acute sign of escalating clinical instability (Garvey, 2015). The healthcare team must investigate and take action to identify the cause of any abnormal data and take corrective action when necessary.

Low blood pressure or hypotension is a very concerning patient finding; it may indicate a late sign of shock or a failure of the heart to function correctly. An infection may cause sepsis or blood poisoning, a life-threatening condition that occurs when the body's response to infection damages its own tissues. Low blood pressure is a critical value in septic patients and may result in the patient's death if not identified and treated aggressively. A low white blood cell count, low body temperature, and low blood pressure are late signs of shock and require rapid interventions by the healthcare team.

Level of consciousness is an essential element of the physical assessment to measure a patient's neurological function. The Glasgow Coma Scale (GCS) is considered the "gold standard" and is an efficient way to accurately measure the patient's neurological responses in three key areas: eye opening, verbal response and motor response. Only 16% of 43 nurses remembered underlying knowledge of the GCS assessment process (Preston & Flynn, 2010). Any restlessness, heightened anxiety, eye pupil changes or signs of confusion are very Important to note and report as this may indicate physiological deterioration. Changes in the patient's neurological status indicate further examination is needed; more questions should be asked, and more data analyzed to understand the severity of findings and identify the underlying physiology resulting in the patient's change.

The human body is amazing and may give clues to underlying function or dysfunction as it tries to compensate. Some clues may be early indicators or warning signs of bodily dysfunction; they may be subtle but can quickly become urgent. If the changes go unrecognized and uncorrected, the patient may continue to deteriorate. For example, a new change in a patient's inability to recognize their spouse is concerning, but if you cannot wake up the patient after shaking and shouting at them, this is *very* concerning and requires urgent action by the healthcare team. Assessment-appropriate interventions may be necessary to save the patient's life and must be implemented quickly.

Josie King

Josie King was a healthy 18-month-old toddler when she experienced 1st and 2nd degree burns from very hot bath water. She was admitted to the pediatric intensive care unit (PICU) at Johns Hopkins Hospital for treatment. She was recovering and healing well. Sorrel King, Josie's mother, noticed that the nurses were frequently pushing the button on the pain pump for Josie. At the time, Sorrel didn't realize the significance of this fact. Josie's condition continued to improve, and she transferred to the intermediate care unit; the physician wrote an order to restrict Josie's fluids (for an unknown reason). Josie cried for drinks when she saw them and sucked furiously on washcloths during bath time. Sorrel noticed Josie's eyes rolling back in her head and was surprised and quite concerned; the nurses told her not to worry—"children do this."

When Sorrel expressed further concern, the nurse placated her with the statement, "her vital signs are stable."

The nurses encouraged Sorrel to go home to get some sleep. When she returned in the morning, she found Josie unresponsive. She cried out to the nurses for help. They gave Josie two doses of Narcan to reverse the effects of the narcotic medication she had received. Thankfully, the Narcan revived Josie. Following this event, Sorrel alerted the physician and nurses that a particular nurse was acting strangely. She argued with that nurse not to give Josie the methadone, but the nurse still administered the medication to Josie. Shortly thereafter, Josie went into cardiac arrest and was resuscitated; she was then transferred back to the PICU for intensive care.

Unfortunately, Josie could not recover from the physiological events caused by the mismanagement of her care. The signs of dehydration and narcotic overdose were not recognized or addressed by the nurses or the physicians. Josie's family was devastated; they made the decision to take their little girl off life support due to the irreversible damage Josie suffered. They visited her bedside one last time, to say their goodbyes to Josie. A tragic and unnecessary death that certainly could have been prevented.

This is an example of the lack of critical thinking and clinical judgment resulting in the end of Josie's short life. A mother's grave concern and anxiety over her daughter's condition were minimized and brushed aside. Not one healthcare provider properly assessed, intervened, or advocated to keep Josie safe. What a tragic and preventable event; the loss of a little girl and devastation for her family.

Ongoing education, skills practice, and clinical competency assessments are crucial to improve nurses' performance in recognizing and responding to deterioration (Considine & Currey, 2015; Mushta, 2018). The education and ongoing training of healthcare team members is essential for high-level team function in mitigating senseless and preventable patient deaths (Subbe & Welch, 2013).

KEY TAKEAWAYS

- *All* patients have the potential to become critically ill.
- Patient deterioration is physiological and observable.
- Observable evidence of clinical instability and patient deterioration frequently occurs from 6–24 hours prior to cardiac arrest.
- Baseline assessment and ongoing patient monitoring and observation are crucial.
- "Speak up" with your concerns and escalate when necessary.
- Be confident in communication with healthcare providers about patient concerns.
- Use **CUS** words to emphasize importance: **Concerned** about . . . , **Uncomfortable** because . . . , **Safety** issue. . . .
- New patient anxiety and confusion for longer than 10 minutes should be investigated.
- Post-surgical patients are at extremely high risk for Failure To Rescue.

CHAPTER 8

RAPID RESPONSE TEAMS AND CRITICAL CARE

Rescue is Just a Call Away!

Mr. Thompson came to the hospital for complaints of shortness of breath; he stated his difficulty breathing had started on the previous day. His chest x-ray showed he had pneumonia, so he was admitted to the medical-surgical unit for treatment and observation. His vital signs were stable, his breathing rate was slightly increased, but he was managing well. Several hours later, Mr. Thompson was found to be sitting forward in his bed and trying to catch his breath; he now had significant difficulty breathing compared with a few hours earlier. He was anxious and restless, his oxygen levels had fallen, and his breathing rate had increased significantly.

The nurse put an oxygen mask on Mr. Thompson, but this didn't seem to improve his breathing or his level of anxiety and distress. Mr. Thompson was not responding to the questions the nurse asked him and began to slump to the side in his bed. The nurse immediately called an internal phone number to activate the Rapid Response Team for help; they arrived in his room just minutes later to assess him and began interventions to help him breathe. Mr. Thompson was immediately transferred to the Intensive Care Unit, where he had a breathing tube place in his trachea and was connected to a ventilator. Several days later, Mr. Thompson's pneumonia and breathing had improved, and he was removed from the ventilator. He was transferred back to the medical-surgical unit for continued care and monitoring.

Rapid Response Teams (RRT) or Medical Emergency Response Teams (MERT) were developed to respond quickly to a deteriorating patient's bedside to evaluate the patient and implement interventions to stabilize the patient as necessary. The creation of the RRT was in response to the devastating crisis identified in the landmark article "To Err is Human"; patients were dying unnecessarily in alarming numbers. This new healthcare team was developed in the early 2000s and adopted by thousands of healthcare facilities across the United States. Hospitals adopted this recommended model of RRT to improve safety in their organizations.

The role and function of the RRT or MERT serves to provide timely and appropriate intervention before a patient suffers a cardiopulmonary arrest. Research shows that 80% of cardiac arrests are avoidable (Quirke, 2011); only 17% of those that suffer cardiac arrest survive to be discharged home. The RRT is expected to arrive at the patient's bedside within minutes of receiving the call for help. The team can assess the patient and perform interventions to stabilize the patient; they communicate directly with the healthcare provider for further interventions if necessary. The RRT actions may include:

- Assessing and stabilizing a patient
- Communicating with the physician
- Performing interventions
- Ordering diagnostic exams
- Transferring patient to a higher level of care (Intensive Care Unit)

The success of the RRT interventions improves drastically if the team is called early in the care of the patient whose condition may be declining. Effectiveness of RRT depends on the nurse recognizing the need to call and activate them for help (Hart, 2016). If the nurse is unsure if patient is becoming unstable and delays calling the RRT, a valuable window of opportunity to intervene early may be lost. The RRT team has been trained to assist and collaborate with the healthcare team to provide necessary care as early and efficiently as possible. To effectively help save patient lives, the bedside nurse must recognize the patient deterioration and call the RRT for help and begin the process of "rescuing" the patient from poor outcomes (Chua et al., 2013).

Nurses report they often feel unsure of themselves and are anxious about calling the RRT; they do not want to "look stupid" and may question if they are making the right decision (Simmonds, 2005). They may fear criticism if the RRT or physician deems activating the RRT was "unnecessary." If nurses are unfamiliar with the patient's condition or do not have a baseline comparison, they may be reluctant to call the RRT. Many nurses do not fully understand the concepts of FTR and miss essential cues of early patient deterioration as we discussed in the previous chapter. They may have difficulty communicating the patient condition to the physician and can be entrenched in the medical hierarchy—all of which prevent or delay activating the RRT (Chua et al., 2020).

The following are parameters utilized by many healthcare organizations to guide RRT activation:

RRT Triggers for Activation—Be Aware!

- Heart rate more than 130 or less than 40 beats per minute
- Systolic (top number) blood pressure less than 90 mmHg (millimeters of mercury)
- Respiratory rate less than 8 or more than 30 breaths per minute

- Oxygen saturation less than 90% (with use of supplemental oxygen)
- Acute mental status changes (confusion, anxiety, restlessness)
- Patient has difficulty speaking clearly or is not making sense
- Airway compromise
- Acute concern about the patient

Nurses are often overwhelmed with an endless list of tasks to accomplish in caring for patients; the workload is frequently a heavy one. In their haste to manage the multitude of responsibilities in caring for patients, they may skip performing patient assessments to save time. Omitting a patient assessment is perilous, as early signs of patient changes may be overlooked. Numerous studies have demonstrated the concerning changes in physiological parameters are both underreported and even disregarded (Panday et al., 2017). The literature demonstrates that many nurses are not able to correctly identify which vital signs were early indicators of patient deterioration (Verrillo & Winters, 2018; Kavanagh & Szweda, 2017). Without nurses having a clear understanding of these key indicators of patient stability, patients are at risk for poor outcomes.

Jackson (2017) noted that the delay in activating the RRT can range from 21% to 56% of all calls, thereby increasing mortality and morbidity. Shearer et al. (2012), found that despite meeting the criteria for activation of the RRT, 42% of the patients did not have the benefit of having the RRT called to assist them during the deterioration event. Healthcare education should involve encouraging nurses and healthcare providers to observe and pay attention to their gut feeling; they should deploy the RRT proactively at the first inkling of trouble rather than taking the standard course of cautiously watching and waiting (Sharek, 2008).

Nurses need a deep understanding of alterations in patient physiology; potential death may be the consequence if appropriate communication and interventions are not taken to mitigate the event. Interpreting the pertinent data points indicating patient stability (vital signs, level of consciousness, critical lab values) is essential to the patient surviving the critical event and returning to a state of health (Rischer, 2022).

The effective utilization of RRT has demonstrated a reduction in events of omission (omitted care), 30-day mortality rates, and decreased length of stay in the hospital (Olsen et al., 2023). In several studies, general care floor or ward nurses report the value of feeling supported and caring collaboratively for patients with the RRT, resulting in improved patient outcomes. Olsen et al. (2022) cite an example of ward nurse and RRT nurse collaborative efforts in their study of the utilization of RRT; they report the ward nurse saying, "We can improve the patient's situation together" and the RRT nurse stating, "I experience that we are saving angels when we arrive." The nurses lowered their shoulders, as they felt that finally somebody has come to offer support and suggestions, and that they are not alone anymore. (Olsen et al., 2022).

Be assertive and call the RRT yourself! Ask about the RRT in the healthcare facility you or your loved one is being admitted to. If you are concerned about your loved one, do not hesitate to activate the RRT by either calling the number the facility has designated for this or insist a nurse calls the RRT. If you do not get a satisfactory response or do not see nurses and doctors taking action, escalate your concern. Find the nurse manager; ask to speak to the nursing House Supervisor or contact the physician yourself.

Critical Care

INTENSIVE CARE UNITS (ICU)

Nurses in the ICU usually have fewer patients to care for during a shift; typically these patients have a higher acuity requiring complex treatments and close observation. In recent years, newly graduated nurses have been hired directly into a staff position in the ICU due to the shortage of qualified nurses. This is a very challenging environment requiring a high level of critical thinking and clinical judgment. These patients can be physiologically unstable due to illness, traumatic events, or critical surgeries. Unfortunately, most new graduate nurses do not yet have the valuable clinical experience of interpreting patient data in a timely manner. Patient outcomes depend on the nurse to accurately observe the patient's status, make rapid decisions, and intervene quickly when necessary.

Approximately 25,000 potentially life-threatening errors occur daily in hospital intensive care units (ICUs). Up to 10 percent of these adverse events involve unintended incidents in airway management; more than half of these errors have been deemed preventable (Needham et al., 2004). Airway management is the process of ensuring the patient has a patent or open airway and can breathe adequately to oxygenate their blood and body tissues. Airway is the first priority in the ABCs of patient resuscitation; without oxygen to the brain, heart and vital organs, life may end within minutes.

When patients are critically ill, they may need to have a breathing tube inserted into their trachea and be connected to a ventilator. Physicians and/or the Respiratory Therapists (in some institutions) may insert and manage this endotracheal tube (ETT) to breathe for the critically ill patient. Patients placed on ventilators are often sedated to relax them and let the machine breathe for them while their body fights to recover and heal. Frequently, the sedated patient may be confused and disoriented due to the medication; they may have their wrists restrained and tied to the bed to prevent the patient accidently pulling the tube out of their throat.

If your loved one is in the ICU, they are usually quite ill and need to be closely observed. The nurse-to-patient ratio here is typically one nurse to two patients. You will probably have quite a few questions about therapies, medications, diagnostic results, and the plan of care. Physician visits in the ICU are not always easy to anticipate as this will vary and depend on their schedule; the physician may visit once or twice daily depending on various factors. Ask your nurse if he/she knows or can find out when the physician is expected to visit so you can be present at the time of the visit. This is your opportunity to obtain information about test results, the plan of care, and the answers to any questions you may have.

EMERGENCY RESPONSE SYSTEM

In the community setting, the emergency response system includes an Emergency Medical Technician (EMT), Paramedic, Flight Teams (nurses, paramedics, respiratory therapists), the Fire Department and the Police Department that make up the Emergency Medical Services (EMS) team. In rural settings, many times there are volunteers with basic medical training to assist the EMS system. The ambulance responds to 911 emergency calls to assist with medical emergencies in most communities and is usually staffed with an EMT and/or Paramedic.

Paramedics and Flight Nurses undergo rigorous training to manage a variety of situations where patients need emergency care. They are trained to assess the airway, breathing and circulation of patients and to prioritize care. This training may include an advanced scope of skills to treat critically ill patients in emergent situations in environments outside of the hospital and in rural locations. These skills require ongoing training, workshops and certifications for emergency-trained personnel to be prepared, up-to-date and relevant in their scope of practice.

The scene or environment in which the EMS team is called to treat a patient may be challenging; calls for emergent help may occur at all times of day or night. These patients requiring immediate care and life-saving interventions may be located in very remote areas where access can be a challenge. A patient may be stuck in a wrecked vehicle and need extrication, found on the side of the highway after being ejected from a vehicle, on a boat at the lake or ocean, or be out in the desert after a four-wheeler or sand buggy accident. Frequently, the patient needs to be moved from a remote location to the rescue vehicle (ambulance or helicopter) to receive higher levels of care in the hospital emergency department or trauma center.

To rescue a patient from respiratory failure, the insertion of a breathing tube (intubation) may be necessary to ensure adequate breathing and oxygenation. Performing the skill of intubation correctly is critical; the tube must be inserted into the trachea (airway) to ensure the oxygen is delivered to the lungs. The trachea or "windpipe" allows the passage of air and vital oxygen to the lungs. The esophagus allows food and liquid to be ingested into the stomach. If the breathing tube is inadvertently placed into the esophagus, or slips out of place, the patient is in imminent danger as the oxygen will be delivered to the stomach instead of the lungs. If the misplacement of the endotracheal (breathing) tube is not recognized and corrected, the patient may suffer anoxia (lack of oxygen) and may suffer subsequent brain damage. Even just a few centimeters can make the difference of the breathing tube moving from the trachea and into the esophagus.

Out in the field or pre-hospital environment, failed intubations occur in as high as 38% of patients intubated by a non-physician, and in as high as 22% of patients intubated by a physician (Crewdson et al., 2017). The pre-hospital environment is "uncontrolled"; many factors contribute to uncertainty in this environment. Lack of adequate lighting, space confinements, sub-standard equipment, and fewer personnel to assist in the procedure may contribute to challenges in securing the patient's airway in the pre-hospital environment. Vigilant care in monitoring and protecting the endotracheal tube position in the trachea is crucial. There are multiple opportunities for the breathing tube to dislodge, especially in the transport environment as the patient is taken to the Emergency Department.

The incidence of failed airways can be as high as 1 in 50–100 in emergency department (ED) and ICU settings. The occurrence of death or brain damage has been reported to be 38 times higher in the ED and 58 times higher in the ICU as compared to the operating room setting with anesthesia (Cook & MacDougall-Davis, 2012). Unplanned extubations happen in over 7% of patients who undergo mechanical ventilation in the ICU; the complications of unplanned extubations result in over $4 billion in healthcare costs (da Silva, 2012).

KEY TAKEAWAYS

- 80% of cardiac arrests are avoidable.
- Early interventions save lives—call the Rapid Response Team early.
- Nurses may hesitate to call the RRT for fear of "looking stupid."
- Call the RRT yourself if you feel concerned about acute patient changes.
- Up to 25,000 potentially life-threatening errors occur daily in ICUs.
- A secured airway is the #1 priority in patient care.
- Correct placement and securement of the endotracheal tube is critical to patient outcomes.
- Failed airways resulting in death or brain damage occur many times more often in the ED or ICU as compared to in the operating room.

CHAPTER 9

THE CRISIS IN NURSING PRACTICE
What the Bleep is Going On?

The American public has ranked nurses as the most honest and ethical professionals for over two decades in a row. Nurses have been voted the topmost trusted profession on the annual Gallup poll, identifying honesty and ethical standards as the valued traits nurses possess. Ranking at the top of the list, by a wide margin, is a very high honor for the nursing profession; they outranked many other professionals including pharmacists, medical doctors, fire-fighters, and grade-school teachers. The code of ethics that influences nursing is founded on truth, honor, dignity, respect for human life, and compassionate care in the goal of restorative health.

The image of a nurse conjures the persona of Florence Nightingale, the lady with the lamp, who saved many lives during the Crimean War in the 1850s. Most people expect the nurse to be caring, compassionate, and a knowledgeable figure associated with illness and injury. Nurses are responsible for managing and directing the healthcare team in caring for their patients. Physicians rely on nurses to assess and monitor their patients and to communicate if a patient's condition changes or deteriorates. Nurses collaborate with the healthcare team, facilitate patient and family education, and are expected to provide a safe environment in which the patient can heal and return to health (Henson, 2020).

Nurse Practice Act

(https://www.ncsbn.org/npa.htm)

Each state in the United States has the duty and obligation to "protect those who receive nursing care"; it is the basis for a nurse obtaining and maintaining a nursing license. Safe, competent nursing practice is grounded in the law as written in the state Nurse Practice Act (NPA) and the state rules/regulations. Together the NPA and state boards of nursing guide and govern nursing practice.

Each state requires a nurse to hold a license to practice nursing in any healthcare setting. The state writes its own regulations to govern the body of nursing practice; this is called the Nurse Practice Act and may vary from state to state. Nurses must abide by the laws of the state where they carry a license and work. Nurses must comply with state licensure renewal requirements, usually every two to three years, which requires proof of continuing education units. The Board of Nursing (BON) for each state will regulate the scope of practice for the levels of nursing, meaning the tasks, procedures or specific job duties will be determined by the BON.

The scope of practice for nurses may vary depending on the level of education obtained; the guidelines are outlined in each state's regulations and bylaws and can be found online on state-specific websites. Each nursing certification or license has specific guidelines outlined and approved by state BONs. Certified nursing assistants, licensed practical/vocational nurses, registered nurses, and advanced practice nurses, such as nurse anesthetists and nurse practitioners, will have a scope of practice identified in the state BON regulations.

Nursing Licensure

The National Council of State Boards of Nursing (NCSBN) is an independent, not-for-profit organization through which nursing regulatory bodies act and counsel together on matters of common interest and concern affecting public health, safety, and welfare. The NCSBN is responsible for the development of nursing licensure examinations utilized to assess the new graduates' level of knowledge. The organization is tasked with ensuring the licensure examination assessing graduate nurses' knowledge is adequate to safely care for patients. The examination does not guarantee the nurse is safe for practice but is a minimum standard of evaluation of the new graduate's level of nursing knowledge.

Recent research demonstrated that the lack of the ability in entry level nurses to apply correct decision-making in patient care situations has contributed to a large number of regularly made errors in patient care. Research cites approximately 60 percent of medical errors were related to the lack of clinical judgment exercised by nurses.

To better assess the new nursing graduate's ability to utilize clinical judgment and practice readiness, the NCSBN revises the National Council Licensure Examination (NCLEX) approximately every three years. As healthcare and technology evolve very quickly, the NCSBN strives to ensure the NCLEX is relevant to current nursing practice. Thousands of surveys are disseminated to nurses in the workforce to assess current nursing practice; the results of these surveys guide the NCSBN in making relevant revisions to the NCLEX.

In recent assessments and evaluations of nursing knowledge and safely caring for patients, it was determined there was a deficit in novice nurses' ability to apply clinical judgment. The NCSBN developed a Clinical Judgment Model to address the identified deficits. This clinical reasoning model contains 6 essential steps a nurse should go through to make correct clinical decisions. Giving safe, relevant, and timely care to patients will improve outcomes and save lives.

1. Recognize cues—what data is relevant and significant?
2. Analyze cues—what potential or actual problem is identified?
3. Prioritize hypotheses—what problem should be acted on urgently?
4. Generate solutions—what actions will help the patient and should be implemented first?
5. Take action—act on what is known.
6. Evaluate outcomes—did the patient's status improve?

The most recent revision of NCLEX—Next Generation NCLEX (NGN) was implemented on April 1, 2023; it is a significant change to past examinations. This examination has been in the creation process since 2018; it contains different styles of questions to assess the newly graduated nurse's knowledge and readiness more effectively for practice. Instead of each question being a "stand alone" question, the new NGN format will present a patient scenario containing six questions pertaining to this patient scenario.

This new format more closely correlates to patient situations the new graduate may encounter when delivering care. Each actual patient in the clinical setting typically has multiple pieces of data that combine to create the patient's health status. Each of those pieces of data should be analyzed separately (i.e., lab values and vital signs) as well as how each data point contributes to the whole of the patient's status. This revised examination should better assess a new graduate's knowledge and ability to apply this knowledge to the patient situation. Ultimately, the integration of the Clinical Judgment Model into nursing curricula should improve the nurses' ability to prioritize patient data and improve outcomes.

"Nurses are expected to be professionally competent and provide high-quality care ethically and clinically" (Numminen et al., 2015). In today's healthcare environment of increasing complexity, emerging technologies, and higher-acuity patients (requiring more nursing care), nurses find themselves in a very challenging climate. Nursing is a highly rewarding yet extremely stressful profession. "In today's complex, fast-paced world of hospital nursing, new graduate nurses face significant challenges when providing patient care and are often unprepared to deal with the realities of practice" (Nielsen et al., 2016). Nielsen mentions new graduates nurses in particular because of the steep learning curve they face in learning to successfully manage the multiple tasks and responsibilities to ensure safe patient care.

Clinical Guidelines

Clinical guidelines are the practices commonly accepted by healthcare practitioners as parameters and guidelines established for safe patient care. Evidence-based research has influenced and guided the modifications in healthcare practices and procedures to improve patient outcomes. Clinical guidelines that were considered the gold standard even a few years ago have been modified, discredited, and abandoned in some instances due to the evidence found in the research.

For example, hysterectomies for "female problems" were recommended to virtually every woman over the age of 45 in the not-so-distant past. These surgeries were highly profitable for the performing physicians. Patients were advised that complications from procedures were "uncommon"; unfortunately, research has proven otherwise. Between 9% and 13% of all hysterectomies resulted in an infection and other serious complications. Venous thromboembolism, genitourinary and gastrointestinal tract injury, bleeding, nerve injury, and vaginal cuff dehiscence (the incision reopens, resulting in protrusion of the bowels) have all been reported after a hysterectomy (Clarke-Pearson & Geller, 2013).

Clinical guidelines for nursing care and healthcare practices may change or be modified when evidence-based research demonstrates a deficit in desired outcomes or when harm may have occurred. Previously accepted and practiced clinical guidelines for procedures (i.e., hysterectomies) have been used in a court of law to exonerate a doctor facing malpractice charges. Even though these clinical guidelines have since been abandoned, defendant-representing attorneys may still provide these procedures as "exhibits" in a court of law as they were pertinent when the care given rendered harm or injury. Following those same guidelines today would have proven physician negligence or even malpractice. It is essential for the medical community to continue investing in research to ensure patients are receiving the safest care possible.

Nurses begin as novices in the profession and can take several years to become competent. It takes time, experience, and the application of critical thinking to develop their skills and clinical judgment to safely care for patients (Benner, 2010). Nursing care requires a complex process and "new" way of thinking for many nurses. The application of learned knowledge to the patient situation involves the "thinking" of the meaning of the patient data collected; this should determine best actions and guide appropriate interventions.

STANDARDS OF CARE

Standards of nursing practice developed by the American Nurses' Association (ANA) provide guidelines for nursing practice and performance. They are the rules or definition of what it means to provide competent patient care. The registered professional nurse is required by law to provide patient care in accordance with what other reasonably prudent nurses would do in the same or similar circumstances. It is critical for nurses to provide high-quality patient care consistent with established standards to promote good patient outcomes.

Basic Nursing Standards of Care

- Provide a safe environment
- Perform a complete admission assessment
- Complete a shift assessment (repeat as patient condition may change)
- Observe patient's ongoing progress
- Interpret a patient's signs and symptoms
- Listen to a patient's complaints and act on them
- Adhere to standardized protocols or hospital policies and procedures
- Act as patient advocate
  - Notify a physician in a timely manner when conditions warrant it
  - Follow a physician's verbal or written orders (unless unsafe)
  - Question a physician's order if it is unsafe
  - Question incomplete or illegible medical orders
  - Question discharge orders when patient condition warrants it
- Follow the manufacturer's recommendations for operating equipment
  - Check equipment for safety prior to use
  - Place equipment properly during treatment
  - Learn how equipment functions
- Communicate effectively with a patient (i.e., ensure effective communication of discharge instructions)
- Seek higher medical authorization for a treatment
- Document in the patient's medical record
  - A patient's progress and response to treatment
  - A patient's injuries
  - Pertinent nursing assessment information (for example, drug allergies)
  - A physician's medical orders

Nurses are expected to perform the following actions for every patient they care for:

- Perform physical assessment
- Interpret physiological findings
- Identify abnormal findings
- Implement interventions to maintain homeostasis
- Notify appropriate healthcare providers of relevant data
- Evaluate the patient after the interventions have been executed
- Document care, data, observations, and communications. "Failure to communicate the nurse's work renders it invisible to others" (Meyer, 2007). Nurses are taught that if it isn't documented, it wasn't done.

Missed nursing care is standard and expected care that is not completed or significantly delayed. A study by McGlynn et al. (2003) identified that 46.3% of patients did not receive recommended care and 11.3% of patients received care that was *not* recommended and was potentially harmful. Recent literature continues to find evidence of the pervasive problem of missed nursing care and the threat to patient safety. The quality of nursing care given to patients directly impacts patient outcomes and is essential for patient safety. Missed nursing care contributes to the frequency of adverse events, critical events, and cardiac arrest (Recio-Saucedo et al., 2018; https://www.hospitalsafety grade.org/).

Challenges Facing the Nursing Profession

NURSING EDUCATION

Nursing education has undergone a metamorphosis in the last three decades. Historically, nursing schools were a clinically based model centered on experiential learning and direct patient care opportunities. Today, nursing schools are academically focused with the majority of the students' time spent in the classroom. Nursing students now receive much less "hands on" learning and direct patient care experience during their clinical rotations; this may lead to poor performance (Saintsing et al., 2011) and contribute to medical errors. Developing nursing knowledge relies upon the opportunity to apply the complex combination of skills and critical thinking to develop the clinical judgment necessary to safely care for patients. (Wangensteen et al., 2012).

Another monumental challenge in nursing education today is the lack of qualified nursing instructors. Most states require the minimum education of a bachelor's degree in nursing (BSN) for clinical and simulation instructors; a Masters in Nursing (MSN) is required to teach most theory or didactic courses. "Nursing schools are unlikely to be able to supply enough nurses to replace retiring nurses, much less alleviate existing gaps. In 2019, *80,407 qualified nursing school applicants were turned away* due to insufficient resources (faculty, clinical sites, classroom space, clinical preceptors, and budget)" (Nursing Solutions, 2021). We cannot seem to find solutions and resources to remedy this concerning situation.

The Bachelor of Science in Nursing (BSN) is the second most difficult bachelor's degree in the country; the bachelor's in engineering is ranked first place in difficulty. Many nursing schools today are "accelerated" with the curriculum designed to go year-round and graduate students in three years versus the traditional four years it takes to earn a bachelor's degree. If you couple these facts together, this will give you an idea of the challenge and potential gaps in knowledge that may occur in any nursing school and in any nursing student.

The COVID-19 pandemic impacted nursing education in a very profound way; many healthcare institutions banned visitors, and unfortunately this included nursing students. In some parts of the U.S., hospitals remained closed to students for many months; in certain areas of California, some student's direct patient care experience consisted of giving injections at vaccine clinics. State Boards of Nursing passed "waivers" to the standard direct patient care hours as well as what clinical experiences were deemed acceptable to meet program requirements. Had this this adjustment not occurred, many students would have had to halt their nursing education until they were allowed back into healthcare organizations to obtain the direct patient care experience. Many nursing students' inability to get "direct patient care" experience resulted in thousands of students graduating from nursing school with very limited or zero direct patient care hours and experiences.

In response to the COVID-19 pandemic, nursing schools shuttered their doors on their campuses and moved the nursing courses to the online environment. Courses such as physical assessment and skills labs were cobbled together to create a learning experience to meet course outcomes and objectives. Many students were doing a health assessment checkoff on a family member or even a teddy bear in an attempt to meet requirements. Though many healthcare institutions recognized this experiential gap and attempted to provide more orientation and onboarding for new graduates, there remains a knowledge and application deficit in these nurses. It is essential for you to understand the impact of this experiential gap on nursing education; it may mean that the nurse caring for you today may have missed opportunities to develop a strong foundation of clinical judgment.

READY FOR PRACTICE?

Interestingly, 90% of nurse educators believe their newly graduated students are ready for practice, but hiring managers in healthcare report that only 10% of new graduates arrive ready for practice. (Wangensteen et al., 2012). Experienced nurses also report that new graduates (novice nurses) are not prepared or ready for practice when they enter the workforce; there is a gap from "theory to practice" that must be identified and closed to protect patient lives.

Unfortunately, it has been found that the education for the health professions does not adequately prepare its students to learn the skills needed to reduce medical errors (Wong, 2020). Despite emphasis on patient safety and programs that have been instituted across various organizations, there has not been much of an improvement in this arena. Only 50% of new nurses feel they are adequately trained to safely care for patients before starting their first job; many feel overwhelmed with the job expectations (Saintsing et al., 2011).

In 2005 (del Bueno), performed a large study of novice nurses with less than one year of work experience, to assess and understand the "readiness for practice" of the participants. This study found that only 35% of these nurses were safe to practice and demonstrated the ability to critically think and act to safely care for patients. What about the other 65% of novice nurses in the work force? How are they caring for patients? (Kavanagh et al., 2017) repeated this study a decade later and found the percentage of nurses that were able to practice safely fell to 23%—a 12% decline. This equates to less than one nurse in four who had the skills to intervene when a patient began to become unstable or deteriorate. Over 5,000 graduates with less than one year of experience were evaluated in this study:

- Only 23% were practice ready and considered "safe."
- 54% were able to recognize a change in patient condition but were unable to manage the problem.
- 23% were unable to recognize meaningful patient changes.

Kavanagh and Sharpnack (2021) repeated this same study and found the percentage of *nurses ready for practice and considered "safe" has fallen to 9%!* This assessment over 15 years of over 10,000 novice nurses' initial readiness for practice demonstrates a shocking situation for patient safety today; we have been trending in the wrong direction for way too long!

The literature reflects challenges and areas of focus identified by researchers concerned with patient safety. Knowledge in the nursing profession doubles every six years and requires the skills to share knowledge with the healthcare team; this requires the integration of technology into education and training programs (Huston, 2013). The Institute of Medicine has stated that nursing education must be current and relevant to the 21st century to ensure the delivery of high-quality patient care (*Future of Nursing*, 2010). As adverse events impact patient safety and patients continue to die unnecessarily in the healthcare system, how do we prepare new graduate nurses and continue to evaluate experienced nurses to recognize patient deterioration (Waldie et al., 2016)?

Nurse educators "must address the brutal facts of failing to prepare graduates; we have a preparation-to-practice gap" (Kavanagh & Sharpnack, 2021). It is the duty of nurse educations to prepare students for safe clinical practice. Instructors who asked Socratic and thought-provoking questions to students in clinical settings, theory class, and simulation experiences were the most helpful in stimulating the development of clinical reasoning in the participants (Herron, 2017). These studies demonstrate that it is imperative for nurse educators to take drastic action to narrow the preparation to practice gap. Nursing education is engaged in teaching "need to know" imperatives to students and essential knowledge concepts, but there remains a critical gap in the application of this knowledge to safely care for patients.

Many students graduate from nursing school having memorized information to pass the test, pass the class, pass the program, and pass the NCLEX to obtain their nursing license. Memorizing information does not prepare a student to become a nurse who is able to critically think. Nurses must be able to recognize the signs and symptoms of patient changes and respond in a timely manner to improve patient outcomes. Competency assessments must be integrated into nursing curriculum to identify knowledge gaps and take action to close these critical gaps. True knowledge acquisition, a deep understanding of patient safety concepts, and the ability to apply this knowledge is vital to safe patient care.

New graduate nurses reported in a survey their top three concerns upon entering the workforce:

- Lacking confidence to be a nurse
- *Fear of harming the patient*
- Fear of being unable to handle the workload (Verrillo & Winters, 2018)

These are very real and valid concerns. Nurse educators have been encouraged by the American Association of Colleges of Nursing (AACN) (https://www.aacnnursing.org/Essentials) to ensure students are held accountable to the mastery of competencies deemed critical for the area of study. Teaching and evaluating a nursing student's ability to perform competently in applying nursing concepts to patient care is essential to patient safety and improved outcomes. By preparing nursing students with experiential learning opportunities to apply the knowledge learned in classrooms to patient care, we are sure to see better patient outcomes.

NOVICE NURSES AND MEDICAL ERRORS

Due to nursing shortages, most vacancies on medical surgical or general care units are filled with new graduate nurses (Bowden, 2018). Many nurses caring for patients on the General Care Floor:

- Are inexperienced and under-skilled
- Have excessive work loads
- Have poor role models
- Lack situational awareness (Hart et al., 2016; Cooper et al., 2010)
- Lack of continuity of care—change in assignments

Novice nurses can feel pressured to perform treatments with which they don't feel comfortable or don't have experience doing; this may contribute to the increased likelihood of making an error. "Novice nurses are coming out of school without adequate preparation for practice in the real world" (Saintsing et al., 2011). Newly graduated nurses are most likely to make mistakes or commit a medical error in their first year of practice (Africa & Shinners, 2020). Research shows that most nurses on the medical/surgical units have less than three years' experience and most of these nurses have less than one year of patient care experience (Hodgetts, 2002). This data is still relevant today as healthcare organizations struggle to employ and retain enough nurses to meet the needs of their patient population.

I have worked with hundreds of nurses and trained and educated hundreds of nurses throughout my career. I can tell you that I believe in my heart that almost all these wonderful people have the best intentions; they sincerely want to be the compassionate caregivers and healers they were trained to be. The education and adequate preparation for clinical practice is severely lacking in many nursing schools and educational environments. Change is essential to protect and safely care for patients.

SUBSTANTIAL NURSING SHORTAGES

The nursing shortage has been an international problem for decades. In the United States, it has been conservatively estimated there are over 340,000 vacant positions in 2020. The average hospital registered nurse (RN) turnover rate is 18.7% while the national vacancy for Registered Nurse (RN) positions in hospitals averages 9%. Every six years the average hospital turns over their entire nursing staff (NSI, 2020). When hospitals are short RN positions, many staff nurses frequently work overtime shifts to care for the patients. Nurses working overtime or more than 40 hours per week are three times more likely to make mistakes.

As reimbursements to hospitals have declined significantly in the last decade, there is constant pressure from hospital administration to reduce costs. Labor costs are the largest expense incurred to operate a hospital; decreasing the number of nurses staffed around the hospital can create big cost savings. "Nursing leaders are challenged daily with balancing nurse staffing levels with financial goals of organizations" (Hart et al., 2016).

Today, hospitals are faced with budget challenges; staff salaries are the largest line-item expenditure and overall cost to run the facility. Hospitals hire travel or temporary nurses on short-term contracts to help fill vacant positions. Traveling nurse contracts are very costly to hospitals; these are meant to be a short-term fix for nursing position vacancies but are frequently renewed due to the ongoing need. These nurses may not be familiar with the hospital personnel and hospital specific policies.

Hospitals can be short-staffed on weekends, holidays, and nights; try to avoid being a patient during these times if you can. The workload of the healthcare team is notoriously heavier on night shifts and on the weekends as there are more patients for each nurse to care for. Nursing shortages are a grave concern; the literature demonstrates that if there are not enough nurses to do the work, the quality of patient care is diminished and may lead to adverse patient outcomes (Aiken et al., 2013). Studies show there are just not enough nurses and many nurses do not have the experience or skills set to mitigate preventable medical error.

The nursing shortage attained equilibrium for a short time in 2008 when many nurses returned to the workforce to help pay their families' bills during the economic downturn. This alleviated the shortage for only a brief time. Today, there are still not enough nurse graduates to fill the vacancies found in healthcare facilities. The anticipated aging workforce heading into retirement is looming on the very near horizon; this trend is already impacting staffing challenges in many organizations.

A safety leader in a large hospital system reflected on the staffing challenges in her facility; she stated, "There are not enough experienced nurses applying for open positions." The recruitment of an experienced nurse averages about three months; this leaves potential gaps in the workforce, creating conditions that may contribute to an unsafe patient environment. This situation creates a very real challenge for hospitals to safely care for their patients; often this may lead to the practice of hiring new graduates into critical care areas (the ICU and the ER). Even with critical care education courses and training offered by many hospitals for these new nurses hired into critical care areas, the new graduate is a novice nurse until they have enough experience to integrate their knowledge into safe patient care.

Nurse staffing shortages have led to multiple medical errors and poor patient outcomes; these include increased medication errors, healthcare acquired infections (HAIs), patient falls and accidents (Kim & and Lee, 2020; Hall et al., 2004). The literature shows a shortage of nurses resulted in an increase in nosocomial infections (obtained by patients from contact in the hospital). Examples you may have heard of are *Clostridium Difficile*, ventilator acquired pneumonia, MRSA, and central line catheter blood infections (Snavely, 2016). Not only does this complicate the patient condition and lengthen the hospital stay, but the annual cost the hospitals incur to treat these patients can exceed $33 billion.

Staffing shortages have been directly correlated to nurses failing to notice a patient deteriorating and poor patient outcomes (Clark & Aiken, 2003). Critically ill patients can be found in all areas of the hospital, not just in intensive care units. These patients need closer and more frequent observations due to the severity of their illness. Without appropriate nurse staffing, nurses on shift may be spread thin and may be caring for more patients than they safely can.

Staffing levels impact the likelihood of nurses missing the signs of deterioration in a patient. When adequate staffing ratios are present, patient adverse events occur at a decreased rate (Ashcraft, 2004; Audet et al., 2018). General ward staffing allows for more patients per nurse than critical care areas in the hospital as these patients are supposed to be "more stable" and require less nursing care. The acuity and complexity of patient care has increased in recent years; patients are sicker than they were in previous years. (Hart et al., 2016; Ryan et al., 2004).

These nurse/patient ratios have been found to contribute to the nurses' ability to anticipate, recognize, and take appropriate action when a patient is becoming unstable. Many facilities utilize an acuity rating system to prepare staffing for each shift. Staffing patterns for acuity would place more nurses in the ICU with fewer patients for each nurse to care for as compared to the medical/surgical floors.

> **Acuity Scale**—(UK Department of Health classification of critical care patients):
> - Level 0: Patients whose needs can be met through normal ward care in an acute care hospital
> - Level 1: Patients who are at risk of their condition deteriorating, or those recently relocated from higher levels of care, whose needs can be met on an acute care ward with additional advice and support from the critical care team
> - Level 2: Patients requiring more detailed observation or intervention, including support for a single failing organ system or postoperative care and those "stepping down" from higher levels of care
> - Level 3: Patients requiring advanced respiratory support alone or basic respiratory support together with support of at least two organ systems. This level includes all complex patients requiring support of multiorgan failure (Ryan et al., 2004).

NURSING EDUCATION CHALLENGES

There are areas of the country with long waiting lists for students to be accepted into nursing programs. Despite the national demand for more nurses, many states with nursing schools face similar challenges and cannot graduate enough nurses to meet the demand. Some state Boards of Nursing (BON) limit or cap the number of students a nursing school may enroll into their programs; regulations may vary from state to state.

A common practice of state BONs is to limit enrollments for new nursing schools establishing a program until there is evidence of student success in passing the national licensing exam—NCLEX. The BON guidelines for a school's curriculum will need to be met and approved; the BON may grant "conditional" approval until the school shows "success" in graduating enough nurses that pass the NCLEX. The school may then approach the BON to have the cap of enrollments extended or lifted to allow more students to enroll in their program. The BON will commonly take several factors into consideration with this decision and may review any documents or data they feel is necessary to make this decision.

It can be very challenging to find enough clinical placement opportunities for students to get their clinical experience in some areas of the country; this limited availability or capacity for clinical sites may impact enrollment opportunities for nursing students. The specialty areas such as Mother/Baby, Mental Health and Pediatrics typically have fewer patient beds and therefore a limited clinical experience opportunity for students. In my experience, we were permitted to bring eight students to a particular clinical site with our instructor, but because of a shortage of employed nurses on the unit to provide oversight of students, we had to limit our student group size to just four students.

Nursing faculty shortages are also a grave concern and directly impact the number of new nurses that could graduate each year. It's challenging to obtain experienced nursing faculty for colleges and universities; the competitive pay nurses can earn at hospitals and benefit packages offered are hard to walk away from. Many schools will onboard, and train experienced clinical nurses who've earned bachelor's or master's degrees to become educators. Engaging students in the classroom with activities, content delivery, and classroom management is a skill that is developed with time and experience.

A Registered Nurse (RN) can take the national examination to obtain a nursing license in the state in which they reside. The nurse may have graduated from a diploma nursing program, an associate in nursing degree program, or a Bachelor of Science in nursing. Historically, there has not been much incentive in salary increases to obtain more education or to earn higher degrees in nursing. A master's degree in nursing is typically required to teach theory or didactics in many states; some states also require a master's prepared nurse to teach in the clinical setting as well. Other state requirements for nurse educators will accept a bachelor's degree in simulation training or to teach in the clinical setting.

NURSING DISSATISFACTION

Many nurses are dissatisfied with their jobs and are leaving the profession altogether. Over 20% of new nurses leave within the first year (Henson, 2020), and approximately 30%–50% of new nurses leave the profession completely or change positions due to job dissatisfaction during their first three years. The reality of the job can be very sobering. Oftentimes, the new graduate may not feel fully prepared to take on the responsibility of patients' lives.

The high nurse turnover and those voluntarily leaving the organization lead to increased workload (Ashley, 2018), causing stress on the remaining workforce. "Since 2015, the average hospital has turned over 89% of its workforce" (NSI, 2020). Nursing doesn't seem to be the life-long profession that it used to be. Studies indicate the current nursing profession has about a five-year lifespan for many nurses (MacKusick, 2010).

In a large survey, Shawn Sefton, Chief Nursing Officer at Hospital IQ (2021) states, of the number of currently working nurses, 90% are considering leaving the profession with 76% of those having fifteen years or more of nursing experience. This exit of experienced nurses is leaving a wide chasm of mentors and role models for the novice nurse. The staffing shortages are real; this contributes to the workload of nurses increasing beyond what is reasonable and safe. Although there are multiple reasons nurses leave the profession, staffing shortages leading to work overload and burnout are a major contributing factor. Poor work environments with limited resources, both in personnel and medical supplies, can lead to job dissatisfaction and contribute to burnout (Aiken, 2013). We saw this occur during the COVID-19 pandemic, where personal protective equipment became very scarce; nurses were re-using supplies that were meant to be single-use items.

Research shows that other contributing factors for nurses leaving the profession are medical illness, returning to school for higher education, work-related injuries, family member needs, and the mental health challenges attributed to moral and ethical dilemmas in the healthcare system today. I remember working in the ICU a few years ago and feeling quite distressed that we were placing a 90-year-old patient on kidney dialysis! Some nurses state they feel the nursing profession is no longer rewarding; the exhaustion of the work overload has taken its toll on them. Unfortunately, higher rates of patient mortality and preventable death have been linked to high nurse turnover.

How can you help? Research shows that healthcare facilities that involve families and loved ones in the care of the patient show better and improved patient outcomes. Familiarity with the patient provides a baseline of a patient's "normal" state. Who knows the patient better than family and loved ones? Who may notice the sometimes-subtle changes in the patient that could indicate early signs of deterioration? Nurses caring for a patient several days in a row become familiar with the patient; they may notice small changes in the patient and alert them to early indications of deterioration (Chua, 2020; Hart 2016). You may request the same nurse to care for you or your loved one if you have built a rapport or sense of trust with a particular nurse. It may not be possible for your request to be accommodated due to the variables involved in staff and patient distribution, but it is worth the ask.

If possible, plan on being present for the nurse bedside shift report; this typically takes place two to three times per day, depending on the length of the shift (usually 8 or 12 hours). This is when the nurses going off and coming on duty meet at the patient's bedside to discuss the care given and the care planned or needed for the patient. This is an opportunity for you to meet the nurse taking over the care, to ask questions, and to share important information with the healthcare team.

AGING WORKFORCE

In 2017, the average age of an RN was 50; 55% of the RN workforce was over age 50 (Snavely 2016). This data translates to over 1 million nurses becoming eligible to retire in the next decade. By 2020, this situation had not improved; the median age of RNs was 52 and nearly 20% of working RNs are aged 65 or older. This exit of experienced nurses is creating a gap of knowledge and experience in the workforce, leaving less experienced nurses as the primary care givers.

The sustainability of health care systems depends on the seasoned and experienced nurses training and mentoring the novice nurses into the profession (Phillips & Miltner, 2015). It is essential for the development of novice nurses to have senior nurses to serve as role models; new nurses need guidance to transition from school to patient care. Nursing is a complex profession; nursing school lays down a foundation of knowledge, but applying that knowledge to practice is challenging. Without the seasoned and experienced nurses working at the bedside with novice or less-experienced nurses, a greater number of patients will be at risk for poor outcomes.

Nursing is one of the most physically challenging occupations; often, it is hard to find the time to eat or hydrate, let alone time to get to the restroom. The role of the nurse frequently involves lifting, turning, and repositioning heavy or obese patients and other physically demanding tasks. Injuries and industry risks (i.e., needle sticks, acquired infections, assault by a patient) are hazards of the profession; occurrences are too frequent despite preventative measures being exercised.

Functional capacity diminishes with age, typically in the mid-40s or older age group. Coordination, balance, and muscle strength typically decline in the aging population; this may leave older nurses at increased risk for injury while caring for patients. Many nurses who work the midnight shift can be sleep deprived; this may result in a decline of psychomotor function, leading to additional risks for workplace injuries to occur (Phillips & Miltner, 2015).

Almost fifteen years ago, the Robert Wood Johnson Foundation recommended healthcare systems employ efforts to retain the high-value experienced nurses in the workforce. Many of these nurses ready for retirement would be a great asset as nursing faculty, instructors, or teachers to augment the current resources at nursing colleges and universities. While this is great in theory, many experienced, older nurses do not have the advanced education of a bachelor's or master's degree to meet the requirements of accrediting bodies for teaching.

NURSE BURNOUT AND COMPASSION FATIGUE

Many nurses state they entered the profession because they want to help other people and have a sense of compassion for humanity; nurses are especially known for their compassion, caring attitude, and helping people (Henson, 2020). Compassion satisfaction is a feeling of fulfillment when caring for others; "making a difference" is highly fulfilling and can contribute to a personal feeling of accomplishment and happiness. While there are many opportunities in the healthcare system to care, help others and contribute to serving humanity, the challenge is real: how does one truly be caring and compassionate while feeling over-worked on a continual basis? How does one be authentically caring and compassionate without experiencing the emotional toll this type of work elicits?

You may have heard the term "burnout" if you have a friend or family member who is a nurse; it doesn't even sound good, does it? The experiences and working environments of nurses can contribute to the feeling of overwhelming anxiety and emotional exhaustion. Nurses find meaning in their work when they can create a meaningful connection to their patients (Goodacre, 2017). When nurses are overworked and don't have time to get to know their patients beyond "Mrs. Jones in room 304," burnout can ensue.

Jarrad and Hammad (2020) discuss the psychological consequences of exposure to stressful experiences and the accumulation of witnessing traumatic events. The healthcare environment is fraught with trauma, shock and human tragedy. Burnout and compassion fatigue is a cumulative process; it may be experienced in any area of healthcare. Although burnout frequently occurs when caring for terminal patients in hospice or palliative care, it can even be found in the maternity department (usually a happy place), when fetal death occurs, or infants are born with life-threatening congenital defects.

I experienced the awful feeling of compassion fatigue when I worked on the oncology floor many years ago; of all patients that need a nurse to listen and show compassion, this is the place. Burned in my memory is the question asked by a 40-year-old patient dying of breast cancer, a single mother of a 16-year-old boy: "Who's going to take care of my son when I'm gone?" I felt like I wanted to sit on her bed and weep with her, but my thoughts of all the tasks I had to get done kept intruding. "I have to check the blood hanging in room 312; I'm overdue in checking the blood sugar in room 325; the patient in room 320 is in the bathroom and needs my help to get back to bed." It's the worst feeling in the world when the internal conflict like this goes on day after day; it can wear you down and impact your sense of well-being.

Nurse burnout has been found to contribute to an increase in medical errors (Halbesleben et al., 2008; Dimova et al., 2018; James-Scotter et al., 2019; Park & Hwang, 2021). A well-functioning and cohesive healthcare team leads to efficiency and job satisfaction; when stress and under-staffing become the "normal" working conditions, members of the healthcare team may exercise poor judgement, increasing the risk and occurrence of medical errors.

Recognition is the first step in implementing any change. Nursing management must be sensitive to the burden carried by many healthcare providers, especially in high-risk areas, i.e., oncology, critical care (both intensive care and the emergency department), pediatrics and neonatal intensive care. Supportive services and crisis management resources should be made available to support nurses undergoing a traumatic experience. A buildup of emotional experiences may occur over time, causing a strain on a person's psychological welfare.

POST-TRAUMATIC STRESS DISORDER (PTSD)

Nurses have been conditioned on the job to compartmentalize the human suffering they encounter every day. It's a profession of compassion, but to survive, we go into automatic mode to get through the experience. When a nurse experiences a traumatic patient situation, particularly when it "hits close to home," it may feel personal and be internalized. The impact of some experiences can affect the nurse in a very significant way, both psychologically and physically.

A case study several years ago gives this example of PTSD: "The nurse in this case was a 36-year-old father of four and had worked in the Emergency Department for three years. He was assigned a 36-year-old male patient who had three children. This patient's van was crushed by an 18-wheel truck on the interstate highway; the accident resulted in multiple broken bones for the patient, a severe head injury for one of his children and the death of another child" (Henson, 2020).

The nurse was deeply affected by this patient and the traumatic accident he suffered; it struck very close to his personal life and his identity as a father. The nurse had difficulty performing his usual job function, frequently forgetting to give his patients their medications or do their prescribed treatments. The result of this type of trauma can cause a stress reaction and impact the nurse's ability to function effectively in the work environment. It is essential for the affected healthcare worker to seek professional guidance when exposed to these types of situations and circumstances.

KEY TAKEAWAYS

- Nursing was voted the most trusted profession for over twenty years.
- Nurses are accountable and responsible for safe patient care.
- Clinical judgment is a vital skill nurses must understand and practice.
- Standards of Care and Clinical Guidelines are commonly accepted recommendations for healthcare practice.
- Know the Standards of Care expected of all nurses.
- *80,407 qualified nursing school applicants were turned away* due to insufficient resources.
- Only 9% of novice nurses are considered safe and practice-ready.
- Novice nurses make more mistakes, contributing to medical error.

- There are critical nursing shortages across the country with over 340,000 vacant Registered Nurse positions.
- 30%–50% of new nurses leave the profession completely or change positions in the first three years.
- The median age of RNs is 52 and nearly 20% of working RNs are aged 65 or older.
- Nurse Burnout is very real . . .
- PTSD can affect nurses and the care they provide to patients.

CHAPTER 10

VITAL SIGNS
Normal or Concerning?

Mrs. Smith had surgery to remove her gallbladder; the surgery was performed without any complications. She was taken to the recovery room to be monitored and was given medication for pain. Shortly thereafter, she was transferred to the medical/surgical floor for further care. The patient was complaining of abdominal pain, an expected finding after this type of surgery. The nurse checked the patient's vital signs and charted Mrs. Smith's blood pressure as 92/56 (a low reading) and a heart rate of 112 (too fast). The nurse gave the patient the prescribed pain medication but did not assess the patient's abdomen or surgical site.

Several hours later the patient's vital signs were taken again with the nurse noting the patient "was a little confused"; she assumed the confusion was caused by the pain medication. The patient's vital signs now reflected a blood pressure of 82/48 and a heart rate of 120 beats per minute; the nurse recorded this data in the patient's chart but did take any further action or communicate any concern. A short time later, a different nurse passing by the patient's room found Mrs. Smith in acute distress; she called for help. Unfortunately, the patient quickly became unresponsive and suffered a cardiac arrest. The hospital's code blue team could not resuscitate her; she was pronounced dead after unsuccessful efforts to save her life.

Vital signs are a set of data points that reflect the state of the patient's health and physiological stability. Vital signs are called "vital" because this data can provide critical indicators of where the patient is on the continuum of health. Monitoring a patient's baseline vital signs and analyzing trends is an integral element in nursing care; a patient's stability can change very quickly. "These parameters should be the most reliable information on the patient's chart" (Mok et al., 2015, Brekke et al., 2019).

As we learned in previous chapters, each vital sign parameter gives pertinent information in assessing the patient's physiological status. Ignoring a single abnormal vital sign or a trend towards abnormal is the easiest way to inadvertently contribute to a patient's death. "When taking observations becomes routine, their importance is forgotten" [Dame Betty Kershaw (2008) Nursing Standard].

Observing changes in vital signs can detect early clinical deterioration and should prompt a nurse or healthcare provider to rapidly intervene if necessary. Multiple studies have confirmed that vital sign abnormalities are the earliest indicators of patient deterioration; these abnormalities frequently occur hours before a cardiac or respiratory arrest. Unfortunately, many studies have found vital sign measurements to be inaccurate, recorded incorrectly, missing in the patient's chart, or recorded and not evaluated by the healthcare team. Abnormal physiological observations are "the most important manifestation of existing or developing critical illness" (Ryan 2004).

Hillman et al. (2005) report that even when hospitals knew they were part of a clinical trial monitoring documentation, staff responses to changes in a patient's vital signs were not adequate. Hodgetts et al. (2002) report that in the 24 hours preceding cardiac arrest, the respiratory rate was recorded in only 27% of cases. The administration of oxygen was documented in only 41% of patients who had a documented fall in oxygen saturation levels.

Vital sign measurements include blood pressure, heart rate, respiratory rate, temperature, oxygen saturation and pain level rating. The healthcare providers order the desired frequency of monitoring of the patient's vital signs; the nurse must also use clinical judgment in assessing the patient's physiological status and stability. For example, if the patient's blood pressure is significantly different than was previously measured, or trending away from the patient's baseline measurements, critical thinking should prompt the nurse to gather more patient data to further assess the patient's condition and stability.

The recording of patients' vital signs on general care floors is considered a routine task and is often delegated to patient care technicians or nursing assistants. These healthcare assistants are trained how to measure and obtain a set of vital signs; they are not trained in how to interpret the data measured, as this is the nurse's responsibility. A patient care technician or nursing assistant may not understand the significance of changes or deviations in "normal" ranges or readings. This knowledge gap and lack of understanding can contribute to lack of urgency in reporting patient changes. As we've discussed, it is very important that these changes be recognized, reported, and acted upon.

Principles of Vital Signs

- Indicators of patient status
- Detect patient changes, may be subtle or obvious
- Baseline measurements provide evaluation and comparison points
- Correlates with other data for overall evaluation
- Aid in diagnoses
- Determine life-threatening situations
- Recognize high-risk patients

Practice Challenges

- Infrequent and/or incomplete monitoring and recording of VS
- Misinterpretation of clinical data
- Delays in reporting significant data
- Guidelines and protocols for monitoring often ignored
- Signs of physiological deterioration overlooked, neglected or poorly managed
- Lack of evidence of appropriate interventions

Four Key Factors Associated with Infrequent Monitoring

- Organization of nursing activities
- Equipment management issues
- Development of nursing observation skills
- Clinical decision-making processes

The following are considered "normal" ranges of vital signs that can be found in nursing and medical textbooks; these are adjusted for age groups. For example, infants and young children have faster heart rates and typically lower blood pressure. Here are the "normal" or average ranges for an adult patient:

- Heart rate: 60–80 beats per minute and regular
- Respirations: 12–16 breaths per minute
- Blood pressure: 120/70 (slight variation in range)
- Temperature: 98 degrees Fahrenheit (slight variation in range)
- Oxygen saturation: 95–100%

Many factors can affect the vital signs; it is the nurse's responsibility to determine what is "normal" for each patient in the given situation. Asking the right questions is part of clinical judgment in determining the patient's status and level of stability; vital signs, pertinent data and patient cues are essential to understand.

- Why was the patient admitted to the hospital and what has occurred since they've been here (did they have a procedure performed or did they have surgery)?
- What is the patient's medical history?
- What are the patient's baseline vital signs; what is normal for this patient?
- What medications is the patient taking that may affect the vital signs?
- Does the patient have other concerning symptoms and assessment data that may indicate instability (confusion or a change in mental status, restlessness, anxiety, agitation, pale or bluish color, cool to the touch)?
- What may be occurring to cause a change in vital signs (is the patient experiencing pain)?
- Is the patient dehydrated; what is the fluid balance (intake versus output)?

It is important to consider the whole clinical picture when assessing the patient. Studies have found that when there is more than one vital sign out of normal range for the patient, the risk of mortality increases (Mok et al., 2015). It is essential to consider all the assessment and patient data in the clinical judgment process; it takes deliberate and thoughtful action in caring for the patient to keep them safe.

Respiratory Rate

Respiratory rate (RR) is counted as breaths per minute. Surprisingly, this vital sign is the most sensitive and *earliest indicator of patient compromise*. Unfortunately, most nurses don't realize the importance of accurately counting the patient's RR; it is the vital sign *most frequently omitted and falsified*! Hogan (2006) gives insight when citing that nurses are taught how to do a skill, but they do not always learn "why" they need to perform the skill. Research shows that approximately 80% of nurses don't count RR; they just write down a number in the chart that is in the "normal range." Allen (2020) found 44% of nurses thought counting RR was not helpful in identifying patients who might be deteriorating. RR reflects changes that occur at the cellular level long before the patient may show signs and symptoms of deterioration. When the oxygen levels are low and the cells can't get enough (supply versus demand), the body "compensates" for this state by automatically increasing the rate of respirations. The respiratory rate is driven by the very sensitive cells attempting to get more oxygen and/or get rid of the excess carbon dioxide (Subbe & Welch, 2013).

If you are concerned about your family member or friend, this is an easy action you can do—count the number of breaths for a full 60 seconds. The normal breath rate for an adult is anywhere from 12–16 breaths per minute. If a patient's breath rate is 20 or greater, this is a cause for concern and reason to closely monitor the patient; more data is necessary to determine the patient's stability. If the patient's RR falls out of the normal range and you are concerned, call for the nurse to share your concern. If the patient's RR is 12, they should be watched closely to ensure it does not slow down to 10 or 8 breaths per minute.

Facts:
- *RR has been found to be best discriminator to identify patients at risk of deterioration.*
- Extreme variations of RR precede adverse events.
- RR trends are integral to early detection of patient deterioration.
- 44% of nurses thought RR was *NOT* helpful in identifying patient deterioration (Allen, 2020).

- RR increases as cellular demand drives physiology to return to homeostasis.
- A decrease in oxygen saturation (SpO2) is a late indicator as compared to the early change in RR.

The following is a quote from a nurse: "Respiratory rate? (giggles) Normal routine? I don't count. It takes up a lot of time. The Sp02 is a more precise indicator of patient deterioration compared to the respiratory rate" (Chua, 2013). You just learned that this nurse's understanding is incorrect; RR is *more* effective in monitoring for early signs of deterioration than Sp02 (Smith, et al., 2011). Garvey (2015) found that nurses chart a RR of 16–20 breaths per minute because "That is what is normal." Your nurse needs your help!

- Alterations in respiratory rate is the most significant predictor of deterioration (Mok et al., 2015).
- Assessment of RR is not considered a priority by many healthcare providers (Cretikos, 2008; Parkes, 2011).
- "Blind spot" occurs when RR checked per protocol every 4 hours as early changes can be missed.
- Change in respiratory status is a leading indicator of adverse patient response to opioid infusion.

In a systematic review of 21 articles measuring Early Warning Systems (EWS) for clinical deterioration, abnormal RR was noted in *every* case (Smith, et al., 2014). EWS were developed to assist the healthcare team in identifying a deteriorating patient. These systems were not created to replace clinical judgment but as an adjunct tool to assist clinicians in their decision making (Panday et al., 2019).

- Monitors record other vital signs automatically; most are not configured to record RR, leading to many nurses "guessing" or just writing down a number.

- RR is often under-recorded or omitted entirely.
- Sentinel events from respiratory depression are caused by wrong dosing of medications 47% of the time and improper monitoring 29% of the time (Joint Commission, 2012).
- Outside critical care areas, few patients are continuously monitored.
- Studies show a poor level of RR recording on the general care floor.
- Health care assistants routinely record VS and do not understand significance of RR.
- Fundamental nursing observations on the sickest ward patients were found to be incomplete.

Emergency Department nurses recorded RR only 29% of the time and depended on the type of presenting problem: Shortness of breath = 91%, Chest pain = 63%, Abdominal pain = 31% (Parkes, 2011).

Nurses and Doctors

- Observed and recorded RR on only 55% of patients.
- Monitored and recorded <50% of scheduled and required vital sign collections.
- Impaired clinical decision-making processes leading to poor critical judgment is all too common.
- Guidelines and protocols for monitoring are often ignored.

Oxygen Saturation

The respiratory cycle consists of both oxygenation and ventilation, inhalation and exhalation. Oxygenation is the process of inhaling oxygen into the lungs which is then distributed to the cells via the circulating blood. Ventilation is the process of exhaling the breath containing the carbon dioxide gases, releasing it from the body. Carbon dioxide is a byproduct of the cellular process; it influences the correct balance of pH in the body and is essential for normal physiological functions. Both adequate oxygenation and ventilation are necessary for homeostasis.

Pulse Oximetry Monitoring

The pulse oximeter is a device to measure the amount of oxygen found in the blood. A decrease in oxygen saturation (SpO2) has been found to be a *late* indicator in patient deterioration. Unfortunately, some nurses believe the Sp02 is a more precise indicator of patient stability than the patient's actual respiratory rate; this is not true (Chua et al., 2013). Observing and measuring the patient's pulse oximetry is a poor substitute for counting the patient's respirations. Unfortunately, this common practice has contributed to the deaths of too many patients.

The Sp02 reading may not be accurate in various patient conditions and should be considered when evaluating the patient. Hemoglobin is the part of the red blood cell that carries the oxygen molecule into the cell; if the patient's hemoglobin is below normal, the Sp02 reading may not be accurate. If the patient's heart muscle is weak, it may not be strong enough to adequately pump the blood with oxygen out to the tissues; this may also affect the accuracy of the oxygen saturation reading. An accurate pulse oximetry signal and accurate reading may be difficult to obtain in a patient with cold extremities and fingers if the sensor is placed there.

Capnography Monitoring

Capnography monitoring or end-tidal carbon dioxide (CO_2), measures the concentration of exhaled carbon dioxide gas during the exhalation process; it measures both the adequacy of ventilation and airflow to the tissues. Measuring the end tidal C02 gas is easily accomplished with a small portable bedside monitor or via the ventilator for patients being oxygenated via an endotracheal breathing tube or a tracheostomy. Physiological changes such as hypoventilation (breathing too slow or too shallow) and apnea (absence of breathing) can be detected early with capnography monitoring allowing rapid medical intervention to "rescue" the patient.

Capnography monitoring is indicated when supplemental oxygen is needed to maintain acceptable oxygen saturation. Any high-risk patient or patients with breathing difficulty should be monitored with a capnography measuring device. The Anesthesia Patient Safety Foundation (APSF) and the Joint Commission recommend observation and vigilance with continuous electronic monitoring for patients in high-risk situations (https://www.apsf.org/search-results/?fwp_search_wp=electronic%20monitoring):

- Receiving any opioid pain medication (due to the high risk of respiratory depression)
- Decreased levels of consciousness
- Patients receiving sedative medications
- Any respiratory impairment
- Head injury
- Known or suspected Obstructive Sleep Apnea

Unfortunately, these best practices are often disregarded or ignored and may result in patient harm or death.

Blood Pressure

The measuring of the patient's blood pressure (BP) is very important; it indicates the perfusion of blood flow to the body tissues and the resistance of flow through the blood vessels. Many

different factors can affect the patient's blood pressure including stress, anxiety, fear, medications, blood volume and various
physiological factors. Understanding the patient's baseline readings and trending the blood pressure measurements may indicate
the patient's place on the continuum of stability.

A patient's blood pressure measurement should be assessed
and evaluated with the other vital signs to get the clear picture
of the patient's status. There is a normal range of blood pressure
as we discussed earlier, but again, this measurement needs to be
individualized to the patient. For example, a patient may have
lost a lot of blood in an accident or during surgery, resulting in
a lower-than-normal blood pressure measurement; a decreased
amount of blood circulating in the body may result in a lower BP
reading. The clinical judgment process in this example would
require the nurse to know the patient's baseline blood pressure
for comparison and evaluation.

If a patient's baseline blood pressure is 150/90 (considered
hypertensive), a blood pressure of 110/70 may be in the "textbook"
normal range but would be considered too low or "hypotensive"
for this patient. Hypotension is the medical term for low blood
pressure; a critical value is a systolic reading of 90 mm Hg or
below. A patient with a systolic reading of 90 or below may be in
critical danger requiring further assessment, close observation,
and frequent monitoring.

Unmanaged hypertension or high blood pressure may put
the patient at risk for a stroke or cerebral bleeding; the fragile
blood vessels may tear or burst under extreme pressure. High
blood pressure has been termed the "silent killer"; many people
don't know they have high blood pressure if they haven't been to
a doctor in a long time. Most patients with high blood pressure
do not experience pain or other indicators of ill health. Occa-
sionally they may complain of a headache, head pressure, or may
experience visual disturbances but may not realize the cause may
be hypertension.

Pain Assessment

"Pain is an almost universally experienced phenomenon," although it is very subjective and may vary from person to person in how it is experienced (Roberts et al., 2021). It is considered the "sixth vital sign" because of the significant information that may signal injury or potential dysfunction in the body. Any pain that is new, becomes worse, or is exaggerated for the presenting situation, should be further investigated, and properly evaluated. Persisting pain may indicate physiological compromise and requires prompt and ongoing assessment.

Pain assessment is essential in understanding a patient's physical and emotional well-being. Pain expression is subjective to each patient; it may vary with gender, culture, and personality. An appropriate pain scale should be utilized to best evaluate a patient's pain. A 0–10 scale (with 10 being the worst pain ever experienced) is appropriate for older children and adults; a happy to sad face scale is useful for young children or patients with language or comprehension barriers. It is important to collect relevant patient pain data such as descriptors and characteristics, endurance of the pain incident, assessment of the area of identified pain (including if the pain radiates to other body areas) and assessing the effectiveness of any treatment given.

The patient story in our next chapter is an example of the importance of the assessment and follow through of the patient's complaint of pain.

KEY TAKEAWAYS

- Observing changes in vital signs can detect early clinical deterioration.
- Inaccurate vital sign measurement and documentation is found in patient charts.

- Nurses and doctors are found to not follow protocols for monitoring vital signs.
- Review "normal" vital sign parameters and implications.
- Respiratory Rate is a vital and earliest indicator of patient decompensation.
- Oxygen saturation or pulse oximetry may not be accurate.
- Capnography monitoring—essential for patients receiving pain medications.
- Pain assessment is vital—new or unusual pain may be concerning.

CHAPTER II

PATIENT ASSESSMENT
Disastrous Consequence of Missed Cues!

Several years ago, Mr. Jones was admitted to the hospital for a right knee replacement, a surgery that went well and without complications. The day following surgery the patient complained of increased pain, and decreased sensation to his right leg and foot. The nurse documented vital signs trending outside of normal, and by evening time, the vital signs continued to deteriorate; no action was taken by the nurse.

The patient's pain continued to persist despite an increase in the amount of pain medication given. The nurse noted Mr. Jones's right foot was cool to the touch and the pulse in the foot had diminished. The nurse notified the surgical resident of the finding; he was not alarmed by this assessment and stated, "It's been like that since surgery." The investigation into this incident found the resident was mistaken. The nurse gave more pain medication to the patient to try and alleviate the pain, but did not communicate this finding to anyone else.

The next morning, the patient's vital signs showed a heart rate of 125 beats per minute and a temperature of 100.9°F; no documentation of an assessment of circulation or sensation of the right leg and foot was found in the patient's chart. The night shift nurse stated in her deposition by the attorney that she did not wake up the patient to assess him during the night because he "was so tired and the doctor was not concerned." At 0600 the orthopedic resident found the patient to have swelling from the right foot up the entire thigh, no sensation, and no pulses could be felt or were obtainable by doppler machine. The patient had demonstrated symptoms of compromised circulation for over 36 hours; the healthcare team egregiously missed this until it was too late. The patient went for emergency surgery, but his leg could not be saved (Zimmerman, 2008). A lawsuit was filed and the patient won the case; no amount of money can replace a leg.

The monitoring of patients is a basic nursing function and expectation; unfortunately, although basic, it is not performed well in many cases (Hogan, 2006) as Mr. Jones's story demonstrated. After basic monitoring, nursing students are taught in the next level of nursing education, the Nursing Process. It has been taught in every nursing school for decades and is the orderly process of prioritizing the care for a patient. "If all nurses were to adopt the primary survey approach (assessment of airway, breathing, circulation, and disability) as the first element of patient assessment, they would be more focused on active detection of clinical deterioration rather than passive collection of patient data" (Considine & Currey, 2015).

The nursing process starts with assessing, noticing any relevant patient data, and should take approximately ten minutes to perform. The nurse should analyze, interpret, and prioritize the patient data to include both subjective and objective information. An action plan of care is created and implemented based on collected data and with the clinical judgment of the nurse. The final and crucial step is evaluating and reflecting on the plan that was implemented: did it have the desired effect or does the plan need to be revised and another intervention executed to accomplish desired outcomes?

The systematic approach of the nursing process is the fundamental guide for delivering quality and safe patient care. It involves the collection of information and critical thinking or using "what is known" by the nurse to prioritize care for the patient. Paramount in this process is identifying the "actual" patient presentation and taking the next step to anticipate a "potential" patient response in the medical situation. This is the process of clinical judgment—applying knowledge from textbooks and classrooms to guide and direct appropriate care to give to the patient. This ability is learned through the process of education, knowledge acquisition and experiential practice. Generally, it takes the novice nurse at least two years of clinical practice to become proficient in care of the patient in the clinical setting (Benner, 1984; Rischer, 2022).

Patient Identification

A fundamental principle of patient care and one of the first things healthcare providers are taught to do is to correctly identify the patient. Correctly identifying the patient is vital to ensure the correct medications are given to the patient and medical treatments and surgery are performed on the right patient. All nurses are taught to check two different patient identifiers before giving medications or performing a treatment on a patient. The consequences of wrong medication, surgeries or treatment deliveries can have harmful outcomes for the patient.

A few years ago, I was a patient myself in the outpatient department of the hospital, undergoing a colonoscopy. As you can imagine, I was very nervous as they would be giving me sedation to put me to sleep for the procedure. Before the physician gave me the sedative in my IV, I looked up at the monitor where they would be viewing my colon and I noticed a name that was not mine on the screen. I asked, "Is that name supposed to be my name?" They replied, "Yes, is that not you?" I answered "No." Then they looked at my hospital identification band, realized their mistake, and changed the name on the monitor to my name.

This error would have resulted in the other patient receiving my colonoscopy results! I also asked them before they gave me the sedation, "Will you be sure to check my respirations and vital signs very closely while I recover and until I wake up?" They gave me a funny look as if they were thinking I was a little kooky but said, "Of course." Knowing what I know about missed observations, interpretation, and action in observing post-procedure patients, I was still very nervous!

60 Second Situational Assessment

The Quality and Safety Education for Nurses (QSEN) published a document to help guide nurses in the process of quickly and efficiently assessing the patient's environment. This process should be performed when the nurse first enters the patient's room. The priority starts with the patient's appearance and level of consciousness; it continues with observing the patient's environment, surroundings, and expected findings.

The visual overview includes any devices, tubes, intravenous lines, urinary catheters, and pumps connected to the patient. For example, if there are IV fluids running, is it the right fluid that was ordered? Is the IV running at the right rate? Is the IV fluid going into the patient's vein or has it infiltrated and is going into the tissues? If a patient is intubated and being mechanically ventilated, there should be suction set up in the room, and an Ambu bag to manually ventilate the patient if necessary. If a patient has had a seizure or is at risk for a seizure, there should be a suction set up in the room. For patients who've had a surgical procedure, the dressing and the surrounding skin should be assessed for any redness, swelling, drainage, or odor.

This quick but efficient process of taking the first minute of the initial patient encounter to assess, assists the nurse in setting a baseline overview of the patient environment and situation.

Being proactive and organized prepares the nurse to respond and act quickly if a patient event should occur.

The Head-to-Toe Physical Assessment

Patient assessment is an expected nursing action to be completed on all patients at the minimum of every shift and as directed by the healthcare provider's orders. Nursing judgment and critical thinking should direct the frequency of the patient assessment and may depend on the patient's condition. Studies confirm the disparity between the physical assessment skills taught in nursing school and what is actually performed by nurses in the hospital setting (Chua, 2019). Many new nurses do not feel confident in their knowledge and skills (Lima, 2014). Other nurses report "I'm too busy to do an assessment." As we learned in previous chapters, physical assessment is an integral part of the patient assessment and is vital to evaluate the patient's status and stability.

As a family member, you may ask the nurse, "How often did the healthcare provider order assessments to be performed on my father?" Or anytime you notice a change, ask the nurse to assess your family member or loved one. It is *not* okay for a nurse to delay an assessment because a patient is sleeping. In nursing school, students are taught to do a "Head to Toe" assessment on a patient to ensure that important patient information is collected and evaluated. The physical assessment should also focus on any system of interest or patient concern (such as the surgical site).

The patient physical assessment should be performed in a systematic order; the following is an example of what you should expect to see performed:

HEAD

- Assessing the patient's mental status is essential. Is the patient oriented to time, place and person or are they confused or agitated or restless? An abnormal level of the patient's blood sugar level or oxygen level may cause confusion, agitation, restlessness, and even non-responsiveness. Oxygen levels and blood sugar levels should be checked immediately with any change in mental status. Disorientation to "time" is often the first change in mental status changes.

- If their eyes are closed, are they easily arousable when you call their name?
- Are the patient's pupils equal and reactive to light when checked with a pen light (mini flashlight)?
- A Glasgow Coma Scale (GCS) is a universal tool to objectively determine any slight change in the patient's level of consciousness; the score ranges from 0–15. For example, an alert and oriented patient that can move all extremities and has their eyes open when awake, is given a score of 15; a patient who is comatose and not responsive earns a score of 3 on the GCS.

HEART

- What is the heart rate? Is it fast or slow?
- Is the heartbeat regular and even or is it irregular (may indicate a skipped or early beat)?
- What are the heart sounds (heard with a stethoscope); is there an audible murmur?
- Can the radial pulse (at the wrist) be felt?
- If radial pulse cannot be felt, can the carotid pulse be palpated at the neck?
- Is the radial pulse the same as the rate heard with the stethoscope on the chest (apical pulse)?

LUNGS

Breath sounds are best heard posteriorly (from the back) and should be listened to in a pattern from left to right and then moving upwards by several inches and side to side to the next section. There should be 8–12 places that are assessed for each breath cycle of inhalation and exhalation. Auscultation in each area should include a full inhalation and exhalation (although you will see healthcare providers move too quickly through this assessment).

- What is the respiratory rate or breaths per minute rate?
- What do the breath sounds reveal? Can wheezing or rattling sounds be heard?
- Are breath sounds equal on both left and right sides?
- Is the patient moving air when they breathe?
- Are they struggling to breathe?
- Can they speak in full sentences or are they trying to catch their breath between words when speaking?

NEUROVASCULAR

- Can the patient move all four extremities?
- Are the hand grasps equal and strong?
- Are the feet able to push firmly on your hands (like pushing the gas pedal)?
- Are the fingers and toes warm; can they wiggle and move them?
- Is capillary refill normal? (Do the nailbeds blanch white when pinched and return to pink within 3 seconds)?
- Is sensation present or unchanged? (Improvement should occur with healing of an injury.)

ABDOMEN

- Is the abdomen soft or firm, flat, round, distended or larger than normal?
- Are there bowel sounds when listening with a stethoscope?
- Is there pain on palpation?
- Is the color uniform or are discolorations noted?

SKIN

- What is the color of the skin overall? Is it pink, pale, bluish, slightly grey, or yellow tinged?
- Is it warm to the touch?
- Is the patient's skin sweaty or clammy?
- Are there any signs of pressure or skin breakdown noted on bony prominences (from not moving around in the bed)?

Pressure Ulcers

The occurrence of pressure ulcers in 2008 was over 374,000 cases and cost over $3 billion to the healthcare system (Den Bos, 2015). More recent evidence based on Medicare claims report that hospital-acquired pressure ulcers contribute to over 60,000 patient deaths each year and cost the healthcare system over $22 billion annually (Padula & Delarmente, 2019). This data reflects hospital patients impacted by pressure ulcers, but research reports a much higher number occurring in patients that reside in long-term care facilities. Studies have shown that pressure ulcers increased over 41% since the COVID-19 pandemic in 2020 (Fleisher et al., 2022). We are trending in the wrong direction for a preventable event costing patients their lives.

The most common areas for pressure ulcers are bony areas such as the heels of the feet, the tailbone, shoulders (if the patient is thin or skinny) and perhaps the hips. If the patient cannot move themselves, they need to be turned on a regular basis; every two hours (minimum) is recommended. If the pressure is not relieved in these areas, the skin can start to break down and open, which can lead to infection. The first sign of pressure is reddened skin; the skin is still intact and has not begun to open yet. Intervention must be taken at the first sign of skin pressure to prevent further breakdown.

It is very important to keep the patient's skin intact; the skin is the first line of defense against infection. The older patient is more prone to skin breakdown due to the natural thinning of the skin as a decrease in collagen occurs with aging. Overweight and obese patients are at high risk for skin breakdown as the tissue's circulation of nutrients and oxygen is diminished. A patient with poor nutrition is at higher risk for skin breakdown; protein and albumin are essential for maintaining skin health and integrity.

High-Risk Patients

John LaChance was admitted to the hospital to undergo shoulder surgery for the repair of a rotator cuff injury. The surgery went well; John was recovering from the surgery and was able to visit with his wife. John experienced nausea, possibly due to the morphine pain pump, and was switched to Dilaudid, an oral opioid pain medication. The nurse told John she could medicate him so he was comfortable and would be able to give him a higher dose of pain medication more often with this pill. John had a history of Obstructive Sleep Apnea (OSA), a condition that causes a change in the quality of breathing and is characterized by periods of time when the patient does not breathe.

The doctors were aware of John's medical history of OSA, but no orders for close observation were discussed or written. His wife went home to sleep thinking he would be comfortable; she would see him in the morning and planned to take him home. Unfortunately, policies for monitoring patients receiving oral opioids may not require electronic monitoring, leaving these patients at risk for unrecognized respiratory depression. This hospital did not require electronic monitoring when patients were taken off IV pain medications. John was considered a "stable" patient as his shoulder surgery went well, and he was expected to go home in the morning; nursing observations were not performed very frequently, and nobody noticed that John had quit breathing.

With the combination of the sleep apnea and the oral opioid pain medication John received, he went into a deep sleep, didn't breathe, and didn't wake up. John's wife was devastated when she was notified that John had died during the night; she didn't understand what went wrong. If John had been continuously monitored, his deterioration would have been noticed; his death most likely would not have occurred.

OBSTRUCTIVE SLEEP APNEA

Sleep-disordered breathing can contribute to a failure to rescue (FTR) incidence and a higher rate of death (Verrillo & Winters, 2018; Kaw et al., 2012). Obstructive Sleep Apnea (OSA) is defined as a complete or partial upper airway obstruction occurring at intervals during sleep. OSA can be present without a patient even being aware they have the disorder. OSA is estimated to impact about 25% of the population, although approximately 90% of those cases have been undiagnosed; the patients have no idea they have this condition.

Patients with OSA have a greater risk of respiratory depression, pauses in breathing and rising carbon dioxide (CO_2) levels that may lead to respiratory arrest and death (Kjorven et al., 2011). When patients are given pain medication or anesthesia, there is less stimulation to breathe and this may result in hypoventilation (breathing too slowly), leading to poor outcomes (Verrillo & Winters, 2018). If a patient has a medical history of sleep apnea (diagnosed or undiagnosed), this may predispose them to respiratory compromise (ECRI, 2017). These patients need continuous monitoring and observation to prevent harm and poor outcomes.

OBESITY INCREASES RISKS

There has been an alarming national trend in the United States of the sharp increase in both overweight adults and children; these individuals are at a much higher risk for disease and illness. Over one in three young adults aged 17–24 are too overweight to meet the requirements to serve in the Unites States military. Of those young adults that meet the weight requirement, many are not physically active and would be challenged to complete basic training for any branch of the military. Unfortunately, many people continue to live unhealthy lifestyles and gain weight, pushing them from the overweight category into "obese" according to healthcare agency guidelines.

The definition of obesity is a Body Mass Index (BMI) over 30 kg/m²; the CDC (2017) has calculated that nearly 42% of adults are obese. This is a significant increase from 30.5% in the year 2000, indicating our national health is headed in the wrong direction. The CDC reports the prevalence of obese children between the ages of 2–19 is 19.7%, impacting about 14.7 million children and adolescents.

Studies show that obese patients have an increased incidence of restriction and obstruction of their pulmonary system due to the extra body weight. This impairment of the mechanics of breathing predisposes these patients to low oxygen states and high carbon dioxide states—an imbalance contributing to respiratory dysfunction and difficulty breathing.

Larger bodies require more oxygen to meet the body's needs, putting the overweight and ill patient in the high-risk category. The greater intra-abdominal pressure caused by increased abdominal girth decreases the lung capacity and increases the risk of aspiration. Increased fat accumulation around the ribs and diaphragm reduces the ability of the chest to expand. Estimates of post-operative atelectasis (partial lung tissue collapse) in the obese patient population is as high as 45%; these patients also have a 40% greater risk for developing pneumonia (Blouw et al., 2003).

Because adipose (fat) tissue is metabolically active, obese patients require more oxygen to meet the body's needs. Adipose tissue also produces more carbon dioxide, which can accumulate in the blood and may contribute to the risk of these patients becoming unstable. The metabolic and physiological demands of the obese body increase the health risks in these patients. It is highly recommended the patient actively attempt to lower their BMI before undergoing surgery or medical procedures if possible.

Healthy lifestyle choices contribute to maintaining a healthy and well-functioning body. Evidence-based research demonstrates that cessation of smoking, controlling blood-sugar levels, and having a normal range body mass index will decrease the patient's risk of acquiring an infection and will improve patient outcomes.

COMORBIDITY

Comorbidity is defined as a patient with the simultaneous presence of two or more diseases or medical conditions. These patients are at higher risk for poor outcomes, more complex clinical management, and increased health care costs. Common medical conditions include diabetes, hypertension, heart disease, kidney disease, and autoimmune disease such as arthritis and gastrointestinal problems. Disease can cause bodily dysfunction, leaving a patient vulnerable to compounded effects when several diseases occur together.

The cost of healthcare for patients with co-morbidities is an economic burden. "In the United States, about 80% of Medicare spending is devoted to patients with 4 or more chronic conditions" (Valderas et al., 2009). There is an immense challenge of medically managing these patients and it can be extremely challenging for healthcare.

The recent pandemic of COVID-19 revealed that patients with preexisting comorbidities were at greater risk of death from this virus. An increased mortality rate was noted with patients who had underlying hypertension, cardiovascular disease, kidney disease and diabetes (Koyyada et al., 2022). Overweight, obese, and older patients were also deemed to be at higher risk of dying after contracting the COVID-19 virus.

VIGILANCE

Vigilance has been defined as "a state of watchful attention, of maximal physiological and psychological readiness, to act, and of having the ability to detect and react to danger" (Hirter, 1995).

For example, the air traffic controller must utilize vigilance to prevent aircraft collisions and fatal accidents; their primary role is accident prevention and keeping passengers safe. Vigilance requires the process of collecting and sorting data, determining the relevance, and attaching meaning to the information received.

Critical thinking is vital in the vigilance process; it means one must anticipate "what might happen" in the given circumstance. Readiness to act is another key component in the process of averting mistakes or potential disaster; this should be an essential element in the training of anyone who is responsible to make decisions when lives are at stake.

Vigilance is part of the "thinking" process behind the actions of the nurse when caring for patients. Assessing a patient's physiological status includes analysis and interpretation of collected patient information such as vital signs, physical assessment findings, laboratory, and diagnostic results. Vigilance is the mental work a nurse must engage in before action is taken. It is the ability to use clinical judgment and critical thinking, to anticipate what may happen, and understand the importance of the cues a patient may display when becoming unstable.

Clinical judgment is the foundation of safe nursing practice. Utilizing clinical judgement is a fundamental skill required to be a nurse; it encompasses almost half of all the tasks a nurse must do to keep patients safe. Patient conditions can change from moment to moment; human bodies are in a constant state of change and do not remain static. Patients must be observed frequently to monitor their status and detect any subtle changes that may occur (Rischer, 2022).

Vigilance is the attention to clinically significant information that is observed by the nurse. It is paying attention and being alert to further cues and signals that may be a warning of impending patient deterioration. The nurse must be prepared to act quickly and efficiently on any changes and concerns to avert a potential adverse event. Florence Nightingale wrote of the importance of a nurse's observation back in the late 1800s; she stated, "The habit of observation is one of the most (if not the most) essential qualities in nursing." Observation is based on knowledge and experience, the application of knowledge learned to the situation at hand (Meyer, 2007).

KEY TAKEAWAYS

- Nursing Process—collecting patient data to create a plan of care, analyzing, interpreting, evaluating patient based on observation and interventions.
- Patients should be identified by two methods every time medications or treatments are given.
- Head to Toe assessment should be done on *every* patient by every nurse or healthcare provider.
- Pressure ulcers contribute to over 60,000 deaths annually and cost $26.8 billion annually.
- 90% of people that have Obstructive Sleep Apnea but aren't aware they have it.
- OSA can be fatal if patients are given opioid medication but are not monitored.
- 42% of adults are obese.
- Obesity contributes to increased risk of morbidity and mortality.
- 80% of Medicare spending is devoted to patients with four or more chronic conditions.
- Patients with comorbidities are at higher risk for poor outcomes.
- Vigilance requires the nurse to observe the patient for clinically significant signs and symptoms.

CHAPTER 12

HEALTHCARE ACQUIRED INFECTIONS
Wash Your Hands!

Alicia Coles, a well-known actress, daughter, and now patient advocate, underwent what was supposed to be a routine surgery for uterine fibroids. She left the operating room with a fever, nausea, and chills—all classic signs of sepsis (blood infection). Her symptoms were dismissed as "a bad response to the anesthesia." Shortly after the surgery, she started having trouble breathing; her abdomen was "hard as cement and flaming red." This is clearly abnormal; it should have alerted the healthcare team to take immediate action.

The physician returned to Alicia's bedside because of her mother's alarm and insistence. As the physician noted the raging infection, he took instruments and an open tray of gauze that had been left at the bedside to poke in the abdominal wound. The patient should have been taken back to the operating room to treat this complication under sterile conditions. Alicia suffered hospital-acquired methicillin-resistant *Staphylococcus aureus* (MRSA), sepsis, and necrotizing fasciitis. She has endured nine surgeries, eleven blood transfusions, and nearly had her left leg amputated due to the complications of the infection.

Alicia left the hospital with a cavernous open abdominal wound that took three years to close. All because of a preventable hospital-acquired infection induced by the surgeon's blatant disregard of basic aseptic principles. Alicia is lucky to be alive, but no patient should have to go through and endure what she did.

In 2018, over 772,000 reported events of HAIs contributed to over 75,000 documented deaths in acute care settings. In response to this shocking data, the Joint Commission took action identifying "Hand Hygiene" as a National Patient Safety Goal (NPSG) to address this egregious situation. The Joint Commission creates a "watch list" of NPSG and distributes this information to the nearly 21,000 healthcare organizations in the U.S. The goals are selected with the intention of high-focus awareness to reduce incidence and patient harm; the ultimate goal is to improve patient safety. The Department of Health and Human Services identified HAIs as a major cause of morbidity and mortality; a significant risk to anyone entering the doors of a healthcare facility. The cost of HAIs has been estimated to run between $142 million and $4.25 billion annually (Schmier et al., 2016).

Health care-acquired infections (HAIs) are an important metric tracked by the Center for Medicare and Medicaid Services (CMS). The CMS program, Hospital Compare, scores facilities based on several categories measuring the level of quality provided by the hospital. Statistics of complications and infections are published and compared with the national benchmark and are available for the public to obtain. The preventable but frequent occurrences of HAIs are frightening!

As we discussed in Chapter 5, when selecting your physician and your healthcare facility, you can and should research the ranking and performance of the healthcare facilities working to decrease HAI occurrences. If you are a patient whose immune status may be compromised by illness or surgery, it is especially important to avoid the possibility of acquiring an infection while being treated at a healthcare facility. HAIs are serious and can be life-altering and may even result in the death of the patient. John Nance (2008) stated, "We're killing eleven patients per hour from nothing but hospital-acquired infections." Though the incidence of HAI decreased over the past decade prior to the COVID-19 pandemic, it is still a significant problem in U.S. hospitals and is again increasing in occurrences. You can find the HAI data in your state. This is tracked by the CDC as they track the HAI type as well as procedure categories in acute care hospitals. I highly recommend finding this data on any healthcare facility where you may need treatment.

Patients at higher risk for HAIs include the older patient and the very young; immune systems in these age groups may not be optimized. Patients with low white blood cell counts are at risk for acquiring infection; their compromised immune system may leave them prone to infections. Critically ill patients needing intensive care are a high-risk category due to the potential failure of an organ system. A patient with a body mass index (BMI) >40 is prone to acquiring more infections of all types as compared to normal-weight individuals. Obesity may impact a patient's ability to fight infection due to the dysregulation of the immune system.

Nutrition plays a major role in overall health including that of the immune system. Malnourished or under-nourished patients are also at risk for increased rates of infection. Physicians historically do not receive much training or education in nutrition during medical school. The body needs protein, healthy fats, nutrients, vitamins, and minerals, all of which are essential for optimal cellular function, healing and health.

The Center for Disease Control and Prevention reported in the 2020 National and State Healthcare-Associated Infections (HAI) Progress Report that recently, ground has been lost in the progress of preventing infections in acute care hospitals. Ventilator-associated infections increased 35%, central-line-associated bloodstream infections increased 24% and an increased incidence of methicillin-resistant *Staphylococcus aureus* (MRSA) was occurring in multiple healthcare settings (https://arpsp.cdc.gov/profile/national-progress/united-states).

Hand Hygiene—Wash, Wash, and Wash!

The very basic principle of infection control and *most effective management of HAIs is hand hygiene* or handwashing and hand sanitizing. Using gloves *does not* mitigate the need for hand hygiene; personnel should wash their hands before and after using gloves. Adequate hand hygiene measures include using an adequate amount of hand hygiene product (alcohol-based gel) or spending an adequate amount of time performing hand washing with soap. The CDC recommends 15 seconds of vigorously rubbing the hands under warm running water, ensuring the areas of the fingernails, between the fingers, wrists and thumbs are included; hands should be dried thoroughly.

Medical personnel are taught very early in the fundamentals course of their education the importance and the proper technique for effective handwashing. *Every* person coming into the patient's hospital room to care for or give assistance to a patient should wash their hands with sanitizing gel or soap and water. This means physicians too! The World Health Organization (WHO) recommends hand hygiene for the following situations:

- Prior to touching a patient (including before touching intact skin)
- Prior to performing a clean or aseptic procedure
- After exposure to or risk of exposure to body fluids
- After touching a patient (including after touching intact skin)
- After touching anything in the patient's environment (including medical equipment)

The COVID-19 pandemic aimed the spotlight on the importance of handwashing for infection prevention. Current research shows healthcare workers still do not implement hand hygiene as directed by the CDC. Nurses have been observed to be compliant with hand washing on average of 42% and physicians at only 38%. In 2019, hand hygiene compliance of all levels of healthcare providers (physicians, nurses, phlebotomists etc.) was estimated at only 47.5%.

Clearly, proper hand hygiene practices have not improved since the pandemic and have actually declined as reported. The lack of proper hand hygiene practice has contributed to the rising rates of hospital-acquired infections since the pandemic. In 2021, four of six infections tracked by the CDC had increased by as much as 14 percent compared to 2020 (Becker's Hospital Review, 2023).

When patients and relatives observe the lack of hand hygiene practice, they are reluctant to speak up and "question staff about their behavior" (Sutton et al., 2019). Patients may also feel vulnerable or too ill to advocate for themselves. Understand that the consequences of not speaking up may endanger the life of your loved one. The CDC has implemented a new campaign, "Clean Hands Count," with the intent of empowering patients and their families to remind healthcare workers of their responsibility in breaking the chain of infection (https://www.cdc.gov/patientsafety/features/clean-hands-count.html?mc_cid=c1189eeca4&mc_eid=5578fa9caf).

Microorganism Transmission

The microorganisms that live in hospital environments can be easily passed between patients by healthcare providers or medical equipment. The failure of healthcare personnel to perform this simple act of handwashing has led to the epidemic of HAIs. Disastrously, this lack of adhering to basics has led to many patients being infected with bacteria or viruses that were not present when they came into the hospital, potentially causing a life-altering impact on a patient's health. The literature discusses that while cleaning and sanitizing the hospital is important, hand hygiene is the easiest and most important task that can prevent HAIs.

It is very important that a patient stop smoking 4–6 weeks prior to elective surgery, as smoking narrows the blood vessels; this prevents nutrients and oxygen from arriving at the surgery site for healing. It is also very important that patients understand and measure their blood sugar levels if they are diabetic or pre-diabetic; blood sugar control before planning a surgery will optimize tissue healing (Ban et al., 2017). After surgery, it is imperative that proper cleaning, dressing changes and "aseptic technique" (keeping the area free of contaminating microorganisms) processes are followed.

HAIs have been a focus of attention in healthcare facilities in recent years and have been categorized to identify specific action plans for reduction and hopeful eradication. Policies and procedures have been implemented to mitigate these potential sources of infections, but unfortunately, HAIs are still occurring at alarming rates.

Any foreign object inserted into a patient's body, including medical devices such as urinary catheters, central line catheters and IV catheters, can introduce microorganisms or become a source of infection. Let's discuss some common sources of infection in the hospital setting to increase your awareness and knowledge.

Catheter Associated Urinary Tract Infections (CAUTI)

A patient's medical condition or surgical intervention may indicate the need for a catheter, a tube inserted into the urethra to drain the urine from the bladder. Approximately 70% to 80% of catheter-associated urinary tract infections are caused by improper insertion technique of the catheter and failure to follow CDC protocols for infection prevention (Balu et al., 2020). The majority of CAUTIs occur in patients who are older, immune compromised, or are female patients due to anatomical differences in the genders. The urethra is shorter in females allowing easier access for bacteria such as the *Escherichia coli* bacteria into the bladder, contributing to infection rates 30 times more often in women than men. *Escherichia coli* is commonly found in the gastrointestinal tract and can easily migrate from the anus to the vaginal opening in female patients.

CAUTIs may cause the patient discomfort, body pain, fever, and increase the length of the hospital stay. Infection can migrate from the bladder into the blood system, spreading the infection throughout the body (sepsis) causing an increase in morbidity and mortality. The best way to prevent CAUTI is ensuring aseptic technique is observed on catheter insertion to decrease the potential introduction of microbes into the bladder. Cleansing around the catheter insertion site daily and when soiled with fecal matter is important to prevent bacterial growth.

Properly securing the catheter to the patient's leg will minimize unnecessary tension on the tubing and help avoid any irritation or trauma to sensitive tissue. The longer the catheter stays indwelling, the higher the risk of infection. The CDC recommends removing the catheter within 24 hours after surgery or as soon as possible; catheters should be discontinued as soon as they are no longer necessary to prevent potential infections.

Surgical Site Infections (SSI)

Twenty percent of all HAIs are surgical site infections (SSI); they are the most common type of infection and cost the healthcare system an average of $3 to $5 billion annually. The Center for Disease Control (CDC) estimates 50% of SSIs are preventable (Barnes, 2018). Surgical sites can get infected if proper procedures to mitigate microorganisms that cause infections are not adhered to. Some pre-surgical protocols include precise cleansing of the surgical site and administering IV antibiotics before the surgery is started.

Preventing SSIs is a dual responsibility of both the healthcare provider and the patient. Physicians and nurses recommended practices include:

- Preparing the skin with antimicrobial cleanser
- Utilization of antibiotics pre-procedure per recommended protocol
- Ensuring sterile technique is utilized prior to and during the procedure or surgery
- Using a surgical safety checklist to ensure safety protocols are followed
- Keeping the patient normothermic (not too cold or too hot)

Signs of infection at the surgical site may include redness, yellowish drainage or discharge, warmth to the touch, increased pain, and swelling of the tissue surrounding the incision. If you notice one or more of these symptoms, report your findings to the nurse or physician as soon as possible.

Central Line Associated Blood Stream Infection (CLABSI)

A central line is a special intravenous catheter inserted into a large vein in the patient; common insertion sites are the internal jugular vein in the neck, the subclavian vein below the clavicle, and the femoral vein in the groin. These are inserted for a variety of purposes such as delivery of blood products, large volumes of IV fluid for rapid delivery, and for medications that may be harmful to blood vessels if delivered peripherally in small veins. Central line catheters are identified as high-risk devices; they require healthcare providers to exercise close observation and infection precautions while caring for the patient. The increased risk of infection from a central line access device is due to the high and rapid blood flow through these large veins leading to the heart.

The incidence of CLABSI had been decreasing by 31% over the five-year period prior to the COVID-19 pandemic in 2020; unfortunately, the rates dramatically increased by 28% by the end of the first half of the year (Fleisher et al., 2022). The micro-organism can enter at the central line insertion site and travel very quickly into the bloodstream, putting the patient's health in jeopardy. The burden of poor patient outcomes ranges from increased length of hospital stay, to increased medical care costs, and to increased morbidity and mortality.

The updated guidelines for central line insertion and care include:

- Provide education and competency assessments for providers inserting the catheter.
- The subclavian vein is considered the preferable site to reduce infection complications.
- The subclavian vein site has a risk for pneumothorax during insertion.
- Ultrasound guidance for central catheter insertion is recommended.
- Use of chlorhexidine-containing dressings is considered "essential practice."
- Replace administration sets every seven days (not sets used for blood, blood products or lipid formulations).
- Apply antimicrobial ointment at the catheter site (Buetti et al., 2022).

Hospital-Acquired Pneumonia (HAP)

Hospital-acquired pneumonia is the most common and deadly infection attributed to healthcare in the U.S. Approximately 65% of HAP cases impacting patients occur outside of intensive care units and occur in non-ventilated patients. Non-ventilated healthcare-associated pneumonia (NV-HAP) occurs in about 1 in every 100 hospitalized patients each year; mortality rates range from 15–30% for hospitalized patients (ECRI, 2022). Most of these patients were found to have comorbidities and clinically vulnerable patient populations. The hospital length-of-stay increased from an average of four days to sixteen days, significantly increasing the cost of care and potential death from HAP (Jones et al., 2023).

Nursing care can positively impact patients' susceptibility to HAP by following evidence-based interventions:

- Elevating the head of the patient's bed between 30–45 degrees
- Deep venous thrombosis prophylaxis
- Peptic ulcer disease prophylaxis
- Daily oral care with chlorhexidine
- Dysphagia precautions (take small bites of food, small sips of fluid, eat slowly, chew food thoroughly)

Ventilator Associated Pneumonia (VAP)

Patients needing breathing support may be placed on a mechanical ventilator (breathing machine); these patients are at risk of developing a lung infection or acquired pneumonia. Ventilated patients account for approximately 35% of the documented cases of HAP. Microorganisms may be found in the ventilator tubing or breathing tube and migrate to the patient's lungs, causing infections. Patients at high-risk of developing ventilator associated pneumonia (VAP) are patients with a history of lung disease, such as chronic obstructive pulmonary disease, or those who have a history of diabetes, alcoholism, smoking, or are obese (Shudaifat et al., 2021).

VAP is a preventable infection; it can be eradicated through following evidence-based protocols. Nurses play an integral role in preventing VAP in the intubated patient population by implementing the strategies noted above and adding these interventions:

- Daily "sedation vacation" and assessing readiness to extubate (remove the tube)
- Keep endotracheal tube cuff pressure between 25 cm to 30 cm H20
- Endotracheal tube with inline suctioning

It is important to be aware of these preventable adverse events for patients; precautions must be taken to improve patient outcomes.

Methicillin-resistant *Staphylococcus aureus* (MRSA)

Almost 120,000 cases of *Staphylococcus aureus* infections and 20,000 related deaths were reported in the U.S. in 2017. This bacterium can become antibiotic-resistant, methicillin-resistant Staphylococcus aureus (MRSA), and is of high concern in the hospital setting. *Staphylococcus aureus* is easily transmitted and can cause skin infections, pneumonia, and infections in the bloodstream. A patient acquiring MRSA is at risk of "invasive infections, sepsis and death" (Kourtis et al., 2019). Without proper handwashing, MRSA can be spread by health care providers; this can be especially dangerous for older or sick patients whose immune systems are weak and may not be able to fight an infection.

Patients housed in long-term care facilities (LTC) or nursing homes are prone to developing MRSA; the spread of this microorganism is commonly found in these environments. Closer quarters, closer contact, and encouraged socialization between patients (to improve psychological health) may contribute to the transmission.

Patients often move between the hospital and the LTC facilities due to serious health issues found in the older population; they may carry the MRSA organism into the hospital with them and spread the infection (Lee et al., 2013). All healthcare staff should follow control measures to mitigate the spread of infections. Following recommended infection control standards is essential to minimize the risk of infection. Infection control "best practices" include following hand hygiene protocols, proper cleaning of hard surfaces and disinfecting practices of medical equipment, utilization of personal protective equipment (PPE), and containment of persons known to be harboring transmittable microorganisms.

Clostridium Difficile (C. diff)

Another bacterium that can be acquired in a healthcare setting without the practice of proper hand hygiene is *Clostridium Difficile*, commonly known as *C. diff*. *C. diff* is a spore-forming exotoxin; it is a toxic bacterium that can be spread from patient to patient via healthcare workers. It can be acquired by touching surfaces such as furniture in the patient's room or medical equipment if this exotoxin is living on the surface. *C. Diff* spores can live up to five months on environmental surfaces if proper cleaning was not performed.

Older patients, sicker patients, and patients with a compromised immune system are more likely to acquire infections. When infected with this bacterium, it can multiply in the intestines of some patients as they take certain antibiotics to treat another infection. An imbalance in the gut microbiome—too little "good bacteria" and an overgrowth of harmful bacteria—may contribute to infections such as *C. Diff*. To determine the presence of *C. diff*, a stool sample is collected and analyzed with a laboratory test.

Clostridium Difficile can cause symptoms such as diarrhea, fever, abdominal pain, and inflammation of the colon; patients may experience more serious symptoms requiring some patients to have part of their intestines surgically removed. While it can be treated by antibiotics, *C. difficile* infections in the elderly and other vulnerable patients are at higher risk for poor outcomes and even death. The CDC estimates that approximately 14,000 to 20,000 deaths occur each year in the U.S. due to the *C. difficile* infection. Unfortunately, the *C. difficile* spores are resistant to alcohol-based hand sanitizers, making it easier for them to spread.

To reduce *C. difficile* infections, the CDC recommends healthcare providers use care in prescribing antibiotics (fluoroquinolones, cephalosporins, ampicillin and clindamycin), using dedicated patient care items and equipment, and utilizing full barrier (gowns and gloves) and meticulous hand hygiene when handling bodily secretions. Hospital disinfectants that contain diluted household bleach will kill the *Clostridium Difficile* spores.

Sepsis

Rory Stuanton was a 12-year-old boy who wanted to be a pilot and was a loving big brother. On a typical Wednesday in gym class, Rory fell while playing basketball and cut his elbow on the gym floor. The gym teacher kindly put on an adhesive bandage to cover the wound, but did not think to first clean the wound. Rory woke in the middle of the night complaining of leg pain; by morning, his temperature had risen to 104 degrees. Concerned, his parents took Rory to the pediatrician. Even though Rory's skin was mottled (indicating decreased blood perfusion) and his vital signs were in the danger zone, the pediatrician did not see any cause for alarm.

The physician dismissed Rory's parents' concerns about their son's illness and stated it was a virus going around that was causing his pain. He was admitted to the hospital to have lab work drawn and to receive intravenous fluids for hydration from the effects of the supposed virus. The lab results demonstrated a critical value showing Rory's precarious and unstable condition; nobody communicated the results to the emergency department. Rory was discharged home despite showing serious signs of critical illness. As Rory's condition continued to worsen and his parents' concern was escalating, they took him back to the hospital on Friday evening. Rory was in septic shock caused by the bacteria that entered his bloodstream through the cut on his elbow. Sadly, Rory's life could not be saved; he died on that fateful Sunday evening.

All infections have the potential to lead to sepsis, a life-threatening infection spreading through the bloodstream systemically throughout the body. Most occurrences of sepsis start with infections acquired outside of the hospital; they can quickly escalate to a life-threatening condition. People at risk for sepsis include patients who:

- Have multiple underlying health conditions
- Have weakened immune systems
- Had sepsis previously
- Have been recently hospitalized with an illness
- Are younger than age one or over age 65

Signs of sepsis requiring immediate medical treatment include:

- High heart rate, low blood pressure, increased respiratory rate (over 20 breaths per minute). *Remember, respiratory rate is the most sensitive indicator between patients that are stable and those at risk of deterioration* (Roney et al., 2015).
- Fever, shivering, or feeling very cold
- Shortness of breath
- Confusion or disorientation
- Extreme pain or discomfort
- Clammy or sweaty skin
- Mottled skin (bluish-red, lace-like pattern)

The incidence of sepsis ranks particularly high in patients in the hospital's intensive care units. "More than 30 million cases of hospital-treated sepsis are estimated to occur every year worldwide, with 5.3 million patients dying from sepsis" (Markwart et al., 2020). Patients that develop sepsis while in the ICU have longer lengths of stay and a higher mortality rate. It is essential the infection prevention protocols are strictly adhered to for these critically ill patients.

Sepsis may lead to major organ dysfunction as the bacteria ravages and wreaks havoc on the patient's body. Organ failure is the end result of a disruption of blood flow or perfusion to the vital organs due to the body's compensatory mechanisms. Failure of one or more organs may occur, impacting the kidneys, the gastrointestinal system, the liver, the brain, the blood system, and the heart. If a patient does not receive early treatment when sepsis begins, it may progress to impact more than one organ system (multi-system organ failure); this may result in the patient's death.

KEY TAKEAWAYS

- *Insist anyone entering the patient's room must wash their hands!!!*
- Over 772,000 reported events of HAIs contributed to over 75,000 documented deaths in 2018.
- Hand hygiene is the single most effective way to decrease hospital acquired infections.
- In 2019, hand hygiene compliance of all levels of healthcare providers (physicians, nurses, phlebotomists, etc.) was estimated at only 47.5%.
- Any invasive procedure should be performed under aseptic technique to prevent bacteria from contaminating the body.
- Patients at high risk for infection are older and younger patients, patients who are immune compromised or malnourished, and patients who smoke.

- Urinary catheters, central lines, ventilators, and surgical sites may cause infections.
- MRSA: 120,000 cases and 20,000 related deaths reported in the U.S. in 2017.
- 14,000 to 20,000 deaths occur each year in the U.S. due to the *C. difficile* infection.
- All infections have the potential to lead to sepsis.
- Over 30 million sepsis cases occur annually.
- 5.3 million patients die from sepsis each year worldwide.

CHAPTER 13

DIAGNOSTIC ERRORS
Missed Opportunities & Fatal Outcomes

Alice, a healthy 15-year-old, tells her own story of how she almost died in November 2021. It all began one weekend with abdominal cramping, chills, a low-grade fever, and vomiting. The intense abdominal pain led her to the Emergency Department, where she was found to have low blood pressure, an elevated heart rate, and an elevated white blood cell count. Alice's abdominal pain worsened; she was given IV fluids and transferred to another hospital for further care as the doctors weren't sure what was wrong with her.

The family's pediatrician told Alice's parents to ask the physician to rule out appendicitis; the physician refused to order a sonogram of her abdomen as "appendicitis pain would be in the right lower abdominal quadrant" and Alice's pain was all over her abdomen. Alice's parents also asked for antibiotics to be administered, but the physician said this was a viral infection and antibiotics were not indicated. Alice's intense pain was ignored by the healthcare team; she was only given Tylenol for the excruciating pain she was experiencing. Finally, Alice's father called the hospital administrator to insist on an x-ray, which finally revealed the culprit—a perforated appendix that was leaking toxins into her body; this is why she was feeling pain across her abdomen and why it was not localized just to the right lower quadrant.

Alice was taken to surgery to remove her appendix; surgical drains were placed to get rid of the toxic fluids draining in her abdomen. She spent a week in intensive care recovering from what could have ended her life—a missed diagnosis. Her mother did research after this horrifying series of events and found research by Dr. Prashant Mahajan, who found up to 15% of appendicitis diagnoses were missed. Approximately half of appendicitis cases do not fit into the "classic" signs category (https://www.cnn.com/2022/12/15/opinions/appendicitis-misdiagnosis-girls-tapper?mc_cid=c1189eeca4&mc_eid=5578fa9caf).

Diagnostic errors impact thousands of patients each year during interactions with healthcare systems. Estimates of patients who have been injured by missed or incorrect diagnoses range between 40,000 and 10 million (Newman-Toker et al., 2020). According to a large autopsy study by Leape et al. (2002), approximately 40,000 to 80,000 deaths per year were caused by diagnostic error. In 2020, ECRI reported in 10% of autopsies, diagnostic errors may have contributed to the patient's death. After reviewing medical malpractice claims, Giardina et al. (2022) reported that most diagnostic errors resulted from failure to diagnose, delay in diagnosing, or wrong diagnosis.

It is estimated that over 70% of a patient chart consists of laboratory data and test results (Verna et al., 2019). Graber et al. (2012) define diagnostic errors as a diagnosis that was unintentionally delayed, or a wrong test ordered; they occur not only in unusual patient conditions but in common diseases such as asthma. Diagnostic errors include a "deviation from generally accepted performance standards" (Giardina et al., 2022). Examination results which are misinterpreted, a lack of follow-up on abnormal results received, or the absence of ordering an examination when it would have been prudent to do so are classified as diagnostic medical errors.

A missed or delayed diagnosis may contribute to the patient not receiving the treatment they need, leading to poor patient outcomes, patient harm and even death. The range of impact on patient outcomes can depend on various factors such as medical conditions and the diagnostic examination. For example, a missed diagnosis of an aortic dissection can result in a patient's death within minutes; but a delayed diagnosis of colon cancer by several months may not have a direct impact on the patient's outcomes.

Diagnostic errors are wide ranging and are not specific to any area of healthcare; they occur in primary care physician offices, hospitals, emergency departments (ED), and ambulatory care centers. Patients in the emergency department (ED) are more likely to experience a diagnostic error. The ED is one of the most challenging clinical settings due to the fast-paced environment requiring rapid life and death decisions. The Agency for Healthcare Research and Quality reported in a systemic review, December 2022, "1 in 18 ED patients received an incorrect diagnosis, and as a result, 1 in 50 suffered an adverse event, and 1 in 350 suffered permanent disability or death."

The top five most serious misdiagnosed conditions identified as contributing to almost 40% of patient harm were: stroke, myocardial infarction (heart attack), aortic aneurysm/dissection, spinal cord compression/injury, and venous thromboembolism. "Mistakes in judgment, lack of knowledge, and lapses in vigilance or memory" (Baartmans et al., 2022) may occur more frequently in this fast-paced environment (emergency department) where quick decisions need to be made.

Mr. Peters, a 48-year-old man, is a common example of a case of a missed diagnosis. He presented to his doctor's office with complaints of a history of rectal bleeding. His physician completed a limited sigmoidoscopy; the test was negative and did not identify any cause for the bleeding. The patient continued to have rectal bleeding and reported this to his physician; the doctor gave him reassurance because of the negative examination done previously. Almost two years later, the patient again presented to his doctor's office; this time with a notable 30-pound (14 kilogram) weight loss.

The patient was admitted to the hospital; further testing showed that the patient had advanced-stage colon cancer with metastasis to the liver. Upon review of his medical records, the physicians concluded that the cancer could have been curable in the early stages when the patient first reported his concerns of rectal bleeding. This unfortunate missed diagnosis was attributed to the substandard medical care this patient received. The doctor should have ordered further testing when the patient continued to have rectal bleeding despite a negative examination.

"Among the general public, doctors get the benefit of a huge halo effect. We routinely accept their diagnoses as being accurate, even though studies have shown that anywhere from 10 to 20 percent of diagnoses are delayed, missed, or altogether incorrect" (Schlacther, 2017). In order for patients to receive high-quality care, physicians must be comfortable with "not knowing" everything and be willing to reach out to a professional colleague who has more experience in the area in question.

Unlike errors such as wrong-site surgery or medication errors which are a "systems" type of error, a diagnostic error often involves a physician who failed to report, act on, follow up or treat abnormal examination results. Most medical training programs do not have a special course or curriculum on diagnosis (Graber et al., 2012). Healthcare education should include an emphasis on high alert diagnoses i.e., "do-not-miss-diagnosis," a process to rule out "worst-case scenarios," and "life or limb threat" to better prepare healthcare providers entering the profession (Al-Khafaji et al., 2022).

Human factors play a large role in missed diagnosis types of medical error; faulty reasoning and cognitive bias have been found to contribute to these situations. Cognitive bias is a thought process that filters information through personal experience; this can skew the interpretation of the data and how healthcare providers make decisions and take action.

Human characteristics of emotion, mood, sleepiness, distracting thoughts, physician-patient incompatibility, or "dislike" can influence diagnostic errors (Al-Khafaji et al., 2022). "Physicians are well aware of diagnostic errors, but there is a general tendency to perceive that such errors are made by someone else, someone less careful or skillful" (Graber et al., 2012).

The degree of experience and the level of personal and professional accountability may contribute to the doctor being vigilant in examining diagnostic results. Physicians have been trained to help people and save lives; they are human and don't like to make mistakes. Most physicians really want to help their patients and certainly don't intend to cause to any patient harm by either an action or lack of action.

The medical community agrees the issue of diagnostic error is a very distinct problem in the realm of patient safety. A survey of 6,000 physicians stated that diagnostic errors are preventable (Graber et al., 2012). Despite advancing technologies, studies have found diagnostic patterns of error continue to occur and include failure to recognize an urgent situation; failure, or delay to consider a diagnosis; failure, or delay to follow up on abnormal test results; and delays or missed consultation requests (Baartmans et al., 2022; Giardina et al., 2022).

As we've discussed, diagnostic errors are preventable. After patient examinations are performed and results obtained from diagnostic tests ordered, the physician must be vigilant in following up to obtain the results and plan the treatment process. The right treatment depends on the right diagnosis derived from diagnostic examination results. Focusing on methods to identify and reduce the incidence of diagnostic error is essential in eradicating unnecessary patient harm and death. Systems-level solutions must be implemented on a global level to address this healthcare crisis.

How Much Can One Family Take?

Sue Sheridan shares the story of her family's suffering and tragic experiences with her son and with her husband. The healthcare system failed her family on two separate occasions, diagnostic errors that could have prevented catastrophic outcomes. Cal was a healthy newborn who began to turn yellow with jaundice at just a few days of age. Unfortunately, a bilirubin test was not ordered; this PKU test only cost 36 cents at the time. Sue was "assured" she was an over-concerned "first-time mom." Due to the untreated and extremely high bilirubin level, Cal suffered brain damage and now has significant Cerebral Palsy and is hearing and visually impaired. This was preventable; Cal could have grown into a normal child had his bilirubin been checked and treated. His symptoms of jaundice certainly pointed to this potential problem but was unrecognized and ignored by the nurses and physician, leading to life-altering damage.

When Cal was four, Sue's husband Pat was diagnosed with a tumor at the base of his skull. Pat underwent surgery to have the tumor removed; they were told the tumor was benign. Six months later the pain returned; his new brain scan found a tumor the size of the surgeon's fist. Unfortunately, this tumor was cancerous. Later, Sue found out the initial pathology report transcribed 23 days after the first surgery described the tumor as malignant. Nobody notified the physician, and the physician did not follow-up; this report got filed without the doctor ever seeing it. Sadly, Pat passed away a short while after they discovered the second tumor.

Very few countries have implemented strategies to reduce these events that may lead to poor patient outcomes; minimal if any effort has been made to discuss the frequent occurrences of diagnostic errors with physicians or healthcare institutions. Most patients are unaware that diagnostic errors and reporting mistakes even happen (Verna et al., 2019). This is why it is essential for you to ask the doctors, nurses, and healthcare professionals what examinations and tests have been ordered and when to expect the results. Don't assume that because you haven't heard anything about the results that they are normal; "no news is good news" is not always true. Be proactive and follow up to get your results if you have not been notified in a timely manner. If the examination results are not normal or are out of range, ask what the specific treatment plan and follow-up will be. Nobody is going to care about this more than you do; you have a right to know this information to make informed decisions about your health.

KEY TAKEAWAYS

- Between 40,000 and 10 million patients have been injured by missed or incorrect diagnoses.
- 40,000 to 80,000 deaths per year have been caused by diagnostic error.
- 10 to 20 percent of diagnoses are delayed, missed, or incorrect.
- One in 18 patients visiting the Emergency Department received an incorrect diagnosis.
- A survey of 6,000 physicians stated that diagnostic errors are preventable.
- The top 5 most serious misdiagnosed conditions contributing to almost 40% of patient harm are:
  - Stroke
  - Myocardial infarction (heart attack)
  - Aortic aneurysm/dissection
  - Spinal cord compression/injury
  - Venous thromboembolism

CHAPTER 14

HIGH RISK MEDICATIONS
Which Ones Can Kill You?

Emily's Story

Emily Jerry, a beautiful blonde two-year-old, her daddy's "little angel," was diagnosed with a brain tumor when she was just 18 months old. The physician told her family that this was a treatable and curable cancer. Grievously, Emily lost her life when a pharmacy technician filled her intravenous bag with more than 20 times the recommended dose of sodium chloride. In the process of receiving her last chemotherapy treatment, Emily awoke from her nap grabbing her head and moaning that it hurt. She started crying and screaming, "Mommy my head hurts, MY HEAD HURTS!" A few short hours later, Emily was placed on life support with irreversible brain damage; she died three days later. An excess of sodium chloride causes severe dehydration of the neuron cells in the brain; left untreated this leads to intracranial hemorrhage (bleeding in the brain). Emily's father learned that pharmacy technicians at this hospital did not need any training or a license to work in the job of preparing IVs. The technician later reported she doesn't know why she made the error; she did not know that the high concentration of sodium chloride could cause cellular damage and death.

Medications may be prescribed to patients for many different reasons. There are over 6,000 medications (and probably more now as you read this); it is extremely difficult for a healthcare provider to know and understand all the possible medications available. Healthcare providers have access to drug reference resources to identify recommended dosages, contraindications, and potentially harmful side effects. What used to be a very large resource book, the Physician's Desk Reference, is now contained on hospital computers and many apps for smart phones. Many institutions have medication carts with a computerized system containing a drug formulary where the information about the medication can be found; this provides easy access for the nurse to find essential drug information while at the patient's bedside.

Medication can be given by different routes such as orally, intravenously, subcutaneous injection, intramuscular injection, rectally, and topically. Medications may take effect and be absorbed at different rates depending on the route they are administered. For example, a pain pill given orally may take 30–45 minutes to take effect and help reduce the patient's pain whereas the same medication if given intravenously may take effect within minutes. The medication's duration of effect usually depends on the route it is administered; pain relief from administration of medication through the IV route generally does not last as long compared to the duration of pain relief from a pain pill.

Intravenous catheters can be inserted into veins to give fluids, blood, medications, and other treatments; it is vital that the intravenous catheter is in the vein and "patent" before any medications are given through it. If the catheter is not inserted properly inside the vein and is placed into the surrounding tissue, or if the IV becomes dislodged and moves out of the vein (infiltration), this can cause trauma to the surrounding tissue.

Infiltration of IV fluid can cause the tissue to swell, become irritated, and feel cool to the touch.

It is crucial to ensure the IV catheter is in the vein prior to injecting any medications or fluids into the site. If the IV fluid has caustic properties, it can cause significant tissue damage if the contents leak into the body tissue. There are medications that can cause permanent destruction of tissue and may result in the need to surgically remove the damaged tissue. In extreme cases, the limb may need to be amputated if the tissue damage is severe enough. Medications given by the IV route have a higher rate of errors than any other route of administration (Al Khawaldeh & Wazaify, 2018). Injecting substances through the vein delivers the contents to the circulation and directly to the heart; caution must be taken to ensure guidelines are followed to ensure best patient outcomes.

The patient and family member should understand what the medication is being given for. Medications are categorized by the action they have on the body; this helps you to understand the expected effect on the body as well as anticipate potential side effects. It is essential for the nurse or healthcare provider to understand the importance of explaining to the patient the essential information about their medications. It is vital that patients understand the indications or purpose and expected effect of the medication, the side effects, the contraindications (when not to take the medication), and the recommended dose and route of administration for the medication. You need to understand more than "it's a pill for your heart." How does it work to help your heart?

The following patient case is a great example of the importance of fully understanding your medications. Ask questions!

Blood Thinners

I'll share with you a sad story of a patient who was given a medication she was told was "for your heart" by a well-meaning nurse.

This medication happened to be a blood thinner and was ordered because the patient had some narrowing of the arteries in her heart. The medication was ordered to prevent a clot from developing in her coronary arteries, which could lead to a heart attack.

Several months later, the woman fell down some stairs and hit her head, immediately bruising the area above her eye, and broke her arm. She was taken to the Quick Care, where the nurse asked about the patient's medical history and what medications she was taking. The patient reported she was taking a "heart pill," thus not raising an "alarm bell" for the nurse or physician. They found out later, this "heart pill" was actually a powerful blood thinner.

The patient started becoming confused and her neurological status began deteriorating; the medical team decided to transfer her to a small rural hospital nearby. This small hospital did not have a CT scanner, but the emergency department physician did not think this examination was necessary for this patient. Several hours later, the patient became more unstable; her neurological status was now deteriorating rapidly. The patient was air-lifted with a flight team to a large hospital where the CT scan showed extensive bleeding in the patient's brain. Unfortunately, there was nothing that could be done to save the patient. She died several hours later; her family was very confused and couldn't understand how and why she died. They obtained an attorney to help get answers and to determine if her death could have been prevented. The family won their lawsuit; the investigation concluded that she was not given the proper medical care at the Quick Care and at the rural hospital.

Blood thinners are very beneficial in the management of various medical conditions, but can cause excessive unintended bleeding. As noted in the story above, any trauma to the patient while taking a blood thinner can have dire consequences. Patients need to be closely monitored when on blood thinning medication and may require laboratory tests to ensure a therapeutic range of thinning versus clotting is obtained. Heparin and Coumadin

(Warfarin) are common medications that require laboratory therapeutic range control for safety. The nurse should instruct the patient to watch for any signs of bleeding when taking any of these medications; the most serious bleeding can occur where it is not visible—in the brain. Changes in the patient's neurological status are concerning symptoms that may indicate immediate help is needed. Blood in the urine, bleeding gums when brushing teeth, dark or black stools, or bruising should be reported. Here is a video link "Staying Active and Healthy with Blood Thinners" by the Agency for Healthcare Research and Quality (AHRQ): https://www.ahrq.gov/patients-consumers/diagnosis-treatment/treatments/btpills/stayactive.html. This link from the AHRQ is a booklet in English (https://www.ahrq.gov/sites/default/files/wysiwyg/patients-consumers/diagnosis-treatment/treatments/btpills/btpills.pdf) and Spanish (https://www.ahrq.gov/sites/default/files/wysiwyg/patients-consumers/diagnosis-treatment/treatments/btpills-esp/btpillssp.pdf). These are helpful tools to explain caution needed for patients taking any blood thinning medications.

Blood Pressure Medications

It is very important for the nurse to measure the patient's vital signs prior to giving the prescribed medications, especially any blood pressure or heart medications. There are four main categories of antihypertensive medications based on the action desired: 1) decreasing water and some salt in the body (a diuretic or "water pill"), 2) relaxing the blood vessels, 3) decreasing the force of the heartbeat, and 4) blocking nerve activity that can restrict your blood vessels. The specific mechanism of action of the medication may also have other effects on your body. For example, if you are prescribed a diuretic, you will probably have to make frequent trips to the bathroom; other antihypertensive medications may lower the blood pressure and the heart rate. It is important for the nurse to measure the BP and heart rate prior to giving these medications to avoid any potential complications.

Although the patient may take this same medication at home with no side effects, the combination of any new medications ordered in the hospital may alter the patient's reaction to their usual medication. Medications can "potentiate" each other, meaning the effect or impact of a medication may be heightened if given together with another medication. This can especially be true if one of the medications is given through intravenous access; this route allows the medication to be directly injected into the bloodstream for a much quicker onset of action and absorption. The oral route for medication administration takes longer for the onset of the action to affect the patient as it must pass through the digestive process and be broken down by the liver or stomach before the medication is released into the bloodstream.

Be alert to the patient feeling "light-headed" or dizzy; this could indicate the blood pressure is too low for this patient (even if the reading is considered normal). Extreme caution must be observed if a patient is feeling dizzy or light-headed; the patient is at risk of falling if they lose their balance. Have them take a few minutes to sit on the side of the bed before rising to adjust and be sure they feel stable to stand. The patient's health condition can impact the patient's vital signs; BP and heart rate may rise, or it may decrease depending on the situation. A physician may order medications, treatments, IV fluids, or procedures that can impact the patient's vital signs. You can check the pulse by placing your fingers on the pulse of the inner wrist on the side of the thumb; if it feels too fast or too slow, call for help. Close monitoring is essential to ensure the patient remains stable.

Pain Medications

Medications prescribed by a healthcare provider to manage a patient's pain can be analgesics (mild), non-opioids, or opioids. Opioids are the strongest pain medication available; they may be prescribed after surgery or for a traumatic event causing bodily injury. Opioid pain medication can be ordered and given to the patient through various routes as we discussed and may depend on the patient's condition. Opioid medication delivery can be administered through an epidural catheter into the patient's spinal fluid where the infusion dose is regulated by a pump. These patients must be very closely monitored.

Oral medications such as pills, lozenges, or lollipops can be given to patients for both acute and chronic pain. An opioid patch delivers medication through the skin and can be an effective treatment for patients experiencing chronic pain. Medication patch application should include a change location of the patch each time it is applied; the patch should have the time and date of application written on it for tracking purposes.

It is very important to make sure the previous patch is removed before applying the new patch to avoid a buildup of the medication in the body. Even though most of the medication is absorbed over the time period that it is on the body, there still is some residual medication that can continue to accumulate in the body and cause unwanted side effects.

Intravenous administration can deliver a small dose of opioid medication given over 1–2 minutes into the vein. Another method of delivery is through an IV pump set to deliver a small continuous dose of pain medication. A patient-controlled analgesia (PCA) pump is another option for opioid pain medication delivery; it is programmed to deliver a set dose of medication and a frequency of dose delivery per the healthcare provider orders. When the patient experiences pain, they can push the button on the pump to receive a dose of the prescribed medication.

PCA pumps are commonly ordered for patients after surgery or a painful medical procedure. Despite an appropriately prescribed dose of medication, patients may have different responses and reactions to these medications. Any patient receiving opioid pain medication is *at risk to experience respiratory depression* and must be closely monitored. It is important that family members should not push the button for the patient. Even if they are groaning in pain, the patient should be alert enough to push the button themselves. Opioid medication can have a cumulative effect and lead to an unintentional "overdose" if not monitored properly.

The most serious side effect of opioid medications is respiratory depression. The patient's respiratory rate must be a minimum of 10–12 breaths per minute to adequately oxygenate the brain, heart, and body tissues. Respiratory rates may decrease quickly or can decrease over time as the opioid medication accumulates in the bloodstream. If the patient is not closely observed and monitored, the respirations may slow enough and result in a cessation of breathing (respiratory arrest). These patients are at great risk and must be treated quickly to reverse the opioid affect if respiratory depression is observed.

Counting the patient's respirations for one full minute is of utmost importance when a patient is receiving opioid analgesics. Spot checking a patient every few hours is not adequate; the patient's ventilation effort, respiratory rate, and oxygenation should be observed often. If unrecognized and left untreated, respiratory depression can lead to respiratory arrest, cardiac arrest, and patient death.

Tissue Plasminogen Activator (tPA)

Blood clots can occur anywhere in the body causing a decreased flow or lack of flow to the tissue. Tissue Plasminogen Activator or "clot buster" is the medication given to dissolve a blood clot that may seriously impact the patient's health. The most dangerous impact of blood clots are ones found in the brain, heart, or lungs; vital tissue in these areas quickly becomes compromised without adequate blood flow carrying essential oxygen. Blood clots in the brain may cause a stroke; a blood clot in the heart can cause a myocardial infarction (heart attack), and a blood clot in the lung can block blood flow and adequate gas exchange of oxygen and carbon dioxide. Each of these situations can lead to serious patient harm or death if not treated rapidly.

If the patient is exhibiting signs of a "brain attack" or stroke, it is paramount for the physician to differentiate the cause; a blood clot or thrombosis, a hemorrhage or bleeding in the brain can both cause a stroke, and the treatment is very different for these diagnoses. The patient will need to undergo diagnostic tests, including a CT scan, to detect or determine the cause of the stroke symptoms. Giving tPA for a blood clot is not without risks; the physician will determine the risk versus benefit of administering this medication. The mechanism of action of tPA can cause bleeding; the most concerning area of bleeding is in the brain and may be fatal. This medication should be used with great caution; watch for signs of confusion and decreased neurological function, as this indicates patient deterioration.

Sedatives

Sedative medications can be administered when the patient is going to have a procedure performed in the hospital or in an outpatient setting. These medications can be prescribed for patients to enhance relaxation for patients who are anxious or are having an extreme anxiety episode. Sedative medications can decrease the intensity of sensation and slow the central nervous system down during a medical procedure. Because of these intended effects, patients must be closely monitored for safety reasons. The patients should not be left unobserved or allowed to get out of bed by themselves until the effects of the medication have worn off. "Studies show that the highest risk of adverse events occurred within 25 minutes of receiving the last dose of IV medication" (Caglar & Kwun, 2011). Examples of sedative medications include the classification of Benzodiazepines, including Xanax, Valium, and Ativan; these are typically longer acting sedatives.

The most concerning side effect of sedative medications is the potential for a decrease in the respiratory rate; if the respiratory rate slows too much, the patient may be at risk for harm.

The patient may not be able to get enough oxygen if their respiratory rate is too slow, and this may contribute to the brain being deprived of oxygen and critical nutrients. Sedatives can also cause the patient's blood pressure to decrease; if the blood pressure is low before the sedative is given, the outcome may cause a serious patient safety risk. Sedative medications may interact with other medications such as pain medications potentially increasing the sedative's effects and placing the patient at risk for harm. Etomidate, Brevitol, and Ketamine are examples of shorter acting sedative medications; they are often utilized in shorter medical procedures requiring the patient to be lightly sedated when they do not need full anesthesia. A patient receiving these kinds of medications needs to be monitored closely until fully recovered and the effects of the medication have worn off.

Elderly patients are commonly prescribed sedative-hypnotic medications to treat insomnia and/or anxiety. Benzodiazepines and sedative-hypnotics may contribute to impaired cognitive function and a poor sense of balance and may increase the incidence of falls in this population (Ragan et al., 2021). Patients and their families should be aware of the risks of these medications and ensure safety precautions are followed, such as assisting the patient getting out of bed or walking, especially at nighttime.

Chemotherapy

Chemotherapy agents may be very toxic to the human body; they were designed to kill cancer cells but may also impact the healthy cells in the surrounding area. The frequently reported side effects of chemotherapy often occur due to the medication harming healthy cells in the vicinity of the cancer cells; gastrointestinal disturbances and hair loss are a few examples. Both oral preparations and parenteral forms of chemotherapy are considered "high alert" medications by the Institute of Safe Medication Practice; this means they can cause significant harm to the patient even if administered correctly (Al Khawaldeh & Wazaify, 2018). These types of drugs can cause serious harm or patient death if they are not properly prepared and administered correctly.

Nurses that administer chemotherapeutic agents go through special training as each of these medications may need special handling during administration. Specialized training for nurses to be certified in chemotherapy administration includes didactic learning as well as a clinical assessment to demonstrate competence. Though the training was deemed adequate, surveys found that nurses admit they don't always comply with protocols learned in their training (Hatatet & Oakley, 2019).

In a study observing 320 inpatients and 334 outpatients receiving chemotherapy, the nurses were found to deviate from protocol in *all* cases observed by at least one step in the complex process. The most frequently missed step was not checking drug preparation time and drug stability prior to administration. Aseptic technique in preparing the chemotherapeutic agents was found to be sorely lacking; wearing gowns, for example, to enhance aseptic technique was not complied with almost 100% of the time. Reported protocol deviations include medications that were not labeled, medications that were mislabeled, wrong drip rates were noted, and wrong diluents were used in some cases (Al Khawaldeh & Wazaify, 2018).

Sorrell (2017) shares a nurse's story of accidentally giving a patient two and a half times the ordered dose of medication; investigation of this error found the cause to be a combination of human error and a systems error. Fortunately, the nurse reported the error, and the physician was able to counteract the side effects of the overdose with another medication. The patient was very sick for the next few weeks; she survived because the nurse reported the incident, allowing the oncologist to treat the patient aggressively with agents to increase her cell counts. The nurse in this case shared her story of the error to help bring awareness to the nursing community; she hopes her transparency helps reduce potential medication errors. By being aware, informed, and asking the right questions, you have the opportunity to protect yourself and your loved ones.

Automatic Dispensing Cabinets

The automated dispensing cabinets (ADC) were designed to help deliver medications in a more controlled manner and to reduce medication errors. They require the nurse to "sign in" with their credentials to retrieve medications for patients. The ADC can be compared to a miniature pharmacy and contains medication prescribed for individual patients as well as medications that may be needed on the nursing unit.

More medications are available than the medication the physician ordered in these cabinet drawers, increasing the potential for medication errors. If the clinician utilizes the "override" option, the nurse has access to multiple medications and may choose the wrong medication; this can result in serious harm to the patient. In one analysis of adverse event reports involving utilizing the "override" option, 77% involved ADCs (ECRI, 2020). The decision to "override" the safety parameters of the ADC, resulted in a tragic patient death at Vanderbilt Hospital in 2017.

Medication errors utilizing ADCs can occur at several points in the process. The drawers in the ADC are stocked and refilled with the medication by a pharmacist or a pharmacy technician. The wrong medication or dose can be placed in the wrong drawer or in the wrong section of the drawer. If the nurse or clinician does not double check the label very closely, a mistake may occur and result in potential harm to the patient. The wrong medication taken from the ADC can be administered if care is not taken and may result in deadly consequences. An example of this type of error and unfortunate event occurred at Vanderbilt Medical Center and is shared in the following chapter.

KEY TAKEAWAYS

- IV catheters must be "patent" and correctly placed in the vein before medications are given.

- It is vital for patients to know what their medications are for, and the expected action and side effects they may experience.

- Blood thinners may cause internal bleeding, the most serious may occur in the brain.

- Blood pressure medications in combination with other medications in the hospital may lower BP unsafely.

- Pain medications may cause respiratory depression (especially if given through the IV route).

- TPA, the "clot buster" may cause excess bleeding; most concerning is in the brain. Watch for signs of confusion and decreased neurological function.

- Sedatives can decrease respiratory rate and blood pressure—patients must be closely monitored.

- Adverse events may occur when the override option is used in Automatic Dispensing Cabinets.

CHAPTER 15

MEDICATION ERRORS
Staggeringly Common!

At Vanderbilt Hospital in December 2017, a patient was admitted with complaints of a head injury. She was taken to the radiology department for a CT scan of her head, an important test to detect any internal bleeding and swelling in the brain. The patient was awake and alert; she shared with the nurse that she was claustrophobic and was anxious about needing to be placed in the CT machine. To calm the patient, the physician ordered a sedative, Versed, to relax the patient for the procedure.

In her haste, the nurse decided to take a shortcut in the medication retrieval process; she utilized the override option in the computerized automatic dispensing cabinet (ADC). This action bypassed the built-in safety function of the ADC and resulted in the retrieval of the wrong medication. Vecuronium, a powerful paralytic, was selected instead of Versed, the physician-ordered sedative medication. The nurse disregarded multiple caution warnings displayed on the ADC and multiple medication safety practices. She ignored the pop-up warnings on the screen of the ADC flashing "Paralyzing Agent"; she did not check the label of the medication, nor did she read the bold letters on the cap of the bottle that said "WARNING: PARALYZYING AGENT."

There is a notable difference between the preparation of the Versed and Vecuronium. Versed is a liquid that can be drawn up directly into a syringe; Vecuronium comes in powdered form and must be reconstituted with sterile water before it can be drawn up into a syringe for injection. The differences in medication preparation should have been another "caution" warning to this nurse. The nurse injected the prepared medication into the patient's IV and proceeded to place her in the CT scanner for the examination.

The patient was not monitored during the CT scan; no pulse oximetry or heart rate monitoring was utilized. Approximately 30 minutes later the CT scan was completed, and the patient was brought out of the machine; it was noted that the patient was not breathing. The emergency medical team resuscitated the patient and was able to get her heart beating again; she was placed on life support and moved to the Intensive Care Unit. Unfortunately, her brain did not receive oxygen during the 30 minutes she was inadvertently paralyzed from the wrong medication; she suffered irreversible anoxic brain injury. Her family made the heart-wrenching decision to remove her from life support several days later. The nurse later told investigators that she was "distracted" by an unrelated conversation with a colleague when she was retrieving the medication. She was charged with reckless homicide for this fatal error that ended this patient's life.

Multiple studies cite medication errors as the most frequently reported medical errors ranging between 35% and 38% of all preventable medical errors (Fernald et al., 2004; Mohammad et al., 2017; Dimova et al., 2018). A study in one hospital in Massachusetts noted 1 in every 20 medications given involved an error or caused patient harm, some with serious and life-threatening results (Mass. Public Health Council Presentation 2017). Patel et al. (2022) cite that 1 in 20 hospital deaths may be drug-related with almost half of the deaths deemed preventable. "Medication errors . . . are not rare events . . . and they compromise the confidence of patients and the general public in the healthcare system. Fortunately, most medication errors are preventable" (American Medical Association, Millenson, 2002).

Some medication errors will not result in patient harm and may go undetected and therefore will not be reported. Medication errors can range from no effect on the patient, to an adverse event requiring medical intervention to minimize the harm to the patient or may result in the patient's death; any error is a serious event. Medication errors include overdoses, underdoses, giving the wrong medication, the wrong dose, at the wrong time, or the wrong route. A medication error where a medication is given to a patient with a known allergy can cause serious harm. Classifications of medications that have been found to have a higher incidence of preventable patient harm include cardiovascular medications, sedative-hypnotics, anti-inflammatory, anti-rheumatic, and medications affecting the central nervous system (Hodkinson et al., 2020).

Antibiotics are a classification of medications that are known to cause potential allergic reactions. Some reactions may be mild or may cause difficulty breathing and potentially anaphylaxis. Typical protocol requires observing the patient for at least 30 minutes after receiving an antibiotic to watch for a potential serious reaction and to ensure they are stable. Inadequately monitoring the patient after medication administration may contribute to poor patient outcomes.

Some medications require a known therapeutic level to be effective and not harmful; a blood sample will be drawn for analysis of the medication levels and may require the medication dosage to be adjusted. For example, if the patient is on a Heparin drip (an anticoagulant), it is very important for the medication level to be within a specified range to prevent blood clotting. If the medication level is too high, it may cause excessive bleeding that could lead to patient harm. A classification of antibiotics (Vancomycin, Tobramycin, and Gentamycin), require blood levels to be monitored and maintained in the correct therapeutic range; this group of medications may cause injury to the patient's kidney function or may contribute to hearing loss.

Safe medication administration is a topic of vital importance; it is imbedded into multiple courses in nursing curricula. Nursing students are taught foundational principles of pharmacokinetics in theory courses such as Pharmacology. Students learn and practice the correct medication administration procedures in the skills laboratory before administering medications to "real" patients. During the students' clinical rotations, correct medication administration should also be reviewed and practiced under the guidance of an experienced nursing faculty. Oversight is essential as students learn to safely apply their skills and follow medication safety protocols in the patient environment.

Nurses must also use critical thinking and clinical judgment to determine if a medication should be or should not be administered to a patient. For example, if a patient's blood pressure is low, a medication for high blood pressure should not be given. This seems like common sense, doesn't it? You would be surprised how many times a nurse is trying to get through the many necessary tasks may not be "thinking" in caring for patients; they may not stop to think or utilize critical thinking and clinical judgment.

Six Rights of Safe Medication Administration

A medication error is preventable if the safe administration process if followed; many errors occur when one of these steps is omitted. To minimize adverse drug events, the following steps should be taken before any medication is administered:

- Right drug
- Right dose
- Right route
- Right time
- Right patient
- Right documentation

According to the National Patient Safety Goals, to correctly identify the patient, the nurse should use two identifiers. As some patients may answer inappropriately, the nurse should not ask the patient, "Are you Mrs. Jones?" Instead, the nurse should ask the patient to: "State your name for me, please." The second identifier should be the patient's identification band confirming their name and medical record number. The nurse should ask the patient if they have any allergies each time they give the patient a medication.

The patients should have an identification band and a separate allergy band (usually it is red) if the patient has any allergies. Medication allergies are listed on the arm band but should also include allergies to latex, paper tape, or any foods causing an allergic reaction. This information should also be documented in the patient's chart. Seafood, peanuts, tree nuts, milk, eggs, and wheat are the most common offenders and may cause anaphylaxis in some people. Anaphylaxis is a dangerous, and potentially life-threatening emergency causing the body to go into shock. Epinephrine pens are prescribed for patients with known extreme allergies to prevent a severe reaction and potential shock.

I attended a nursing conference several years ago to hear Ridley Barron tell the devastating story of his family's car accident that was fatal for his wife and critically injured his seventeen-month-old son. The child survived the car accident and was transported to the hospital for intensive care. Five days later, the boy was accidentally given a critical overdose of an anti-seizure medication, causing his untimely and catastrophic death. Mr. Barron chose to share his experience with healthcare organizations from the patient's perspective to humanize the experience; his hope is to inspire immense changes in healthcare organizations' safety practices. Sharing personal stories of loss can build national awareness of medical error and the shattering effects it has on families; active and open communication can help prevent further tragedies.

Each patient can respond differently to various medications.

Understanding the purpose of the medication prescribed as well as precautions you should be aware of is important for your well-being. Medications the patient takes at home may frequently be continued at the hospital; caution is necessary as there are various factors that may impact the combination of new hospital medications and the home medications.

When some medications are given together, there can be an increased or decreased mechanism of action. For example, if a patient takes a medication to control high blood pressure and is given pain medication after a medical procedure or surgery, the combination of the medications may lower the patient's blood pressure too much. Home medications may need to be adjusted when the patient is in the hospital and receiving additional medications.

Bar-coded medication administration systems are widely used in the healthcare setting today. These were developed and implemented to decrease errors in medication administration. The computerized system helps clinicians match the medications to the physician orders at the patient's bedside. The patient has a bar-code on their identification band to confirm the correct patient has been identified for the medications dispensed. When the system is utilized correctly, medication errors decrease and patient safety increases.

Patients who are being transferred from the intensive care unit (ICU) to a general care floor are at increased risk of medication errors and adverse events. The most common medication errors in these patients are due to the failure to discontinue medications indicated for acute and critical care and restarting the patients' long-term home medications (Bourne et al., 2023). The ICU is typically a very busy environment with acutely ill patients, critical medication administration, multiple medical monitors, and various procedures.

The nursing hospital supervisor is responsible for hospital bed management and may need to move patients out of the intensive care unit to accommodate a more acutely ill patient. Acutely ill patients in the emergency department or a patient that has deteriorated on the medical/surgical floor may take priority and need to be in the intensive care unit. In the flurry of activity of high acuity and prioritization, medication reconciliation can be neglected, errors may occur in discontinuing or restarting some medications (Bourne et al., 2023).

In the transfer of patients to another care area, communication may be lacking between healthcare providers; many will verbalize only what they feel to be important or pertinent. Because of the large volume of documents and records in patients' charts, important information may be overlooked or lost in the data. Nursing staff on the general ward may not be familiar with acute care medications resulting in a lack of questioning the medication list; if the medication administration record indicates a medication is due at noon, for example, the nurse may just administer the medication without realizing it may not be appropriate or necessary outside of the ICU.

Caution must be taken when medications are given to patients. Armed with this knowledge you've learned, you can be a patient safety advocate by engaging with your healthcare team and asking relevant questions. Medication errors can be significantly decreased and even mitigated with everyone working together and sharing pertinent information.

KEY TAKEAWAYS

- One in every 20 medications given involved an error or caused patient harm.
- Up to 38% of preventable medical errors are due to medication mistakes.
- Nurses must use clinical judgment and critical thinking when administering medications.
- Review the six "Rights" of safe medication administration.

- Therapeutic levels of certain medications are essential for patient safety.
- Allergic reactions can be life-threatening; antibiotics are a common offender.

CHAPTER 16

TUBES, DRAINS AND DEVICES
What Can Go Wrong?

Grant Visscher was just 11 days old when he died from a misplaced feeding tube. Little Grant had survived heart surgery right after birth and was doing well. Unfortunately, a nurse misplaced a feeding tube through the baby's nose and didn't realize the tube had perforated his trachea. The milk intended for his stomach began to fill up his lungs. Grant started "blowing bubbles" and turning blue; the nurse called for help, but it was too late; the damage to Grant's lungs could not be reversed. Grant could not be resuscitated and died from this medical error.

There are various types of tubes, drains and devices that are utilized in the hospital to treat patients' medical conditions to improve or restore health. There are inherent risks with any procedure or placement of a device into the patient's body. Unfortunately, related adverse events are common and can result in significant harm to the patient. The physician and nursing staff should explain the purpose, procedure, and potential risks involved with these types of procedures.

Feeding Tubes

When a patient is unable to ingest liquids or food due to various medical conditions, a small diameter tube can be inserted into the patient's stomach to infuse liquid nutrition. For patients who require support for short-term nutritional needs, the feeding tube can be inserted through the nose or mouth and advanced into the patient's stomach. For patients with a long-term medical condition that prevents them from taking nutrition orally, a feeding tube can be surgically inserted through the patient's abdomen into the stomach (gastrostomy tube). Feeding tubes are very beneficial to patients who need liquid nutrition, but these tubes are not innocuous or harmless.

When the feeding tube is inserted through the nose or mouth, the healthcare provider must exercise extreme caution. There are two anatomical openings in the back of the throat that are located within centimeters of each other—the esophagus leads to the stomach and the trachea or "windpipe" leads to the lungs. If the tube intended to go to the stomach with liquid food is incorrectly inserted into the trachea or slips out of place, the nutritional liquid can inadvertently be infused into the patient's lungs. Any foreign substance can be very caustic or toxic to the lung tissue and may contribute to respiratory complications and even death.

In an analysis in Pennsylvania hospitals, more than half of enteral feeding tube misplacements were serious events (AACN, 2018). The complications of a misplaced feeding tube include perforated lung causing a pneumothorax; misplaced into the lung instead of the stomach; coiling of the tube in the throat; and perforation of the gastrointestinal tract or esophagus (Wallace, 2017). The feeding tube can be inadvertently connected to patient devices intended for other purposes that may cause grievous harm to the patient. The Joint Commission has issued several Sentinel Event Alerts due to a feeding tube inadvertently being connected to intravenous tubing and vice versa.

ECRI (Emergency Care Research Institute, 2018) reports several examples of feeding tube errors resulting in patient deaths. Tragically, a feeding tube was misconnected to a ventilator suction catheter, causing the liquid to be infused into the patient's lungs. In another deadly case, the feeding tube was connected to a pregnant woman's intravenous line, directly infusing the liquid feeding into her bloodstream. Sadly, neither the patient nor the fetus survived this catastrophic medical error.

A study conducted in Pennsylvania hospitals over a five-year time period found 166 feeding tubes were misplaced; 137 of these were misplaced into the lungs. This error resulted in 11 patient deaths due to pneumothorax (Wallace, 2015). A pneumothorax is either air or fluid in the space between the chest wall and the lung, causing the lung to collapse. If a pneumothorax is left unrecognized or untreated, it may progress to a tension pneumothorax, resulting in the patient's death.

X-ray confirmation of proper tube placement is the safest method and should be utilized upon initial insertion of the feeding tube. Migration of the tube out of the stomach can occur after insertion; proper tube placement verification is an expected nursing action when caring for these patients. Tube placement must be assessed every four hours and prior to introducing feedings or medication instillation. This may be done by aspirating and testing the pH of the fluid in the tube. A reading of the pH <5.5 is considered "safe"; this range indicates the acidity of the stomach fluid differentiating it from fluid found in the lungs. A concerning study found 88% of nurses are not utilizing evidence-based methods to verify tube feeding placements (Motta et al., 2021).

NOTE: A patient with a feeding tube needs the head of the bed elevated at least 30 degrees. If the head of the bed is lowered to give care such as baths or to change the bed linens, the feeding should be paused or stopped during this time. When the patient is lying flat, there is considerable risk for the patient to aspirate the feeding liquid into their lungs. The healthcare providers must exercise caution during patient care; the patient should be returned to a safe position with the head of the bed elevated to at least 30 degrees after care is provided. Call the nurse immediately if you see the head of the bed too low or flat when tube feedings are infusing.

Nasogastric Tubes (NGT)

Nasogastric tubes may be a necessary medical treatment in some patient situations. A physician may order a nasogastric tube (NGT) to be placed through the nose into the stomach to treat a medical condition. The NGT may be ordered to empty the stomach contents by attaching the tube to low intermittent suction or it may drain to gravity. An NGT may be ordered to instill liquid nutrients and/or medications for patients who cannot eat solid food for short term needs. The nasogastric tube is larger in diameter and is a stiffer plastic than the longer-term feeding tubes mentioned prior.

To ensure the tube is inserted to the correct depth to be positioned correctly to reach the stomach, the nurse will take measurements before inserting the tube. The tube will be used to measure from the patient's nose, around their ear and ending at the bottom of the sternum area, noting the black hashmark on the tube. This measurement or hashmark will denote how far the tube is to be inserted the proper depth into the patient's stomach. The NGT should be securely taped to the patients nose to maintain placement and prevent tube dislodgment. The black hashmark on the tube marking the correct depth should be documented in the patient's chart.

This procedure is not without risk and must be performed with caution and monitored with care. It is very important that every precaution is taken to ensure the tube is correctly placed in the stomach as intended. To confirm placement, it is imperative to follow "best practice" and policy to verify correct placement of the tube; a confirmation of correct placement should be verified with a chest X-ray. No liquid or medications should be instilled into the NGT before correct placement in the stomach is verified.

Between 2005 and March 2011 the NPSA was notified of 21 deaths and 79 cases of harm due to misplaced NG tubes (Medical Protection 2012, NGT Errors). Unfortunately, the NGT can also result in the puncture of a lung if the tube is misplaced (AACN, 2012). Motta et al. (2021) reports that 3.2% of nasogastric/feeding tubes "were inserted into the airway resulting in pneumothorax and death." If a pneumothorax occurs, it is imperative this event is recognized, and urgent action taken to mitigate harm to the patient.

NGTs are contraindicated in patients with a suspicion or confirmation of a basilar skull fracture. These patients may have a disruption in the cribriform plate; this injury may allow the NGT to enter the brain and may potentially cause intracranial perforation. Vocal cord paralysis and harm to the larynx (voice box) due to NGT insertions have been documented in the literature. Wu et al. (2006) reports a patient who suffered a fatal massive hemorrhage caused by the nasogastric tube being misplaced on insertion; it perforated the esophagus and damaged a major blood vessel resulting in the patient's death.

It is common for patients with an endotracheal tube (ETT) to have an NGT inserted to decompress and empty the stomach to avoid aspiration of stomach contents. The NGT may be inadvertently misplaced upon insertion into the lungs despite the presence of an ETT; confirmation of proper placement is essential. An NGT to empty stomach contents may lead to an electrolyte imbalance in these patients; a deficit of potassium and sodium may result in patient complications. It is very important to monitor the electrolyte levels by laboratory examinations every day to ensure the patient is adequately hydrated; electrolyte replacement therapy should be initiated if indicated.

Endotracheal Tubes (ETT)

Endotracheal tubes (ETT) are placed in the patient's trachea (windpipe) when they cannot effectively breathe for themselves, or if the patient cannot protect their own airway due to a decreased level of consciousness or head injury. The insertion of this tube requires skill and experience to place it correctly in the trachea. Emergency medicine physicians, anesthesiologists, paramedics, flight nurses with advanced airway training, and Certified Nurse Anesthetists are healthcare providers trained with the skills to intubate (place an ETT) in a patient.

As we previously discussed, the esophagus (tube leading to the stomach) is located right next to the trachea in the back of the throat. The esophagus is a larger opening than the trachea; it is much easier to inadvertently misplace the tube into the esophagus and miss the intended trachea. If the tube intended to deliver oxygen into the patient's lungs is inserted into the esophagus, the brain and body will not receive the oxygen essential for life. Brain death will occur within minutes if this error is not quickly detected and corrected.

Even if the ETT is placed correctly, it can still easily slip out of the trachea and into the esophagus. The highest priority of the healthcare team managing the patient with an ETT is ensuring the patient's airway remains open and intact; it is vital the ETT remains in the trachea at the right depth of insertion to properly oxygenate both lungs. The gold standard confirming correct ETT placement is a chest X-ray examination after insertion. Outside of the hospital environment, a C02 detector should be utilized to help confirm the proper tube placement. The intubated patient should be electronically monitored, measuring all vital signs, continuous levels of oxygenation, and end tidal C02 levels.

Unfortunately, studies demonstrate that failed intubations (not placing the ETT correctly into the trachea), occur in a high number of cases outside of the hospital. Approximately 20% of field intubations were unsuccessful and over 5% were determined to be mal-positioned upon arrival at the emergency department (Denver Metro Airway Study Group, 2009). The uncontrolled pre-hospital environment and potentially difficult patient situations can contribute to the challenge of securing and maintaining a patient's airway. Factors contributing to challenges in placing the endotracheal tube include facial trauma, blood or vomitus in the patient's mouth and nose, airway swelling (making landmarks difficult to visualize), a short neck, and obesity. Pre-hospital or field intubation should be implemented in patients who are deemed at risk for losing control of their airway, in patients whose respiratory compromise may lead to oxygen deprivation, or when oxygen adjunct devices are ineffective (Gnugnoli et al., 2023).

Mimi Toomey shares the tragic story of her husband Dave Bunoski's death after suffering a cardiac arrest in an ambulance enroute to the hospital. Dave needed a breathing tube placed during this emergency, but the endotracheal tube was mistakenly placed in the patient's esophagus instead of the trachea. Unfortunately, Dave suffered an anoxic brain injury during the fifteen minutes he went without oxygen. His wife was not aware of this tragic event that occurred in the ambulance until she questioned why her husband was still in a coma and on the ventilator four weeks after the cardiac arrest. The pulmonologist finally told her about the error of the ETT misplacement during her husband's transport to the hospital. This is another deadly example of a tragic but preventable medical error; had the misplacement of the ETT been recognized and corrected early, Mimi might still have her husband with her today.

Chest Tubes

Chest tube insertions date back to the time of Hippocrates, where they were utilized to save soldiers suffering trauma to the chest during wartime (Seyma et al., 2021). Today, a chest tube is a minor surgical procedure performed in the hospital by a physician. If a patient is having trouble breathing and is short of breath, a chest

X-ray may be necessary to determine a condition or cause of the patient's distress. The chest X-ray may detect a condition where air or blood has accumulated in the space between the lung and chest wall; it may be medically necessary to insert a chest tube to treat the patient's condition.

Chest tubes can be inserted in emergent conditions or during procedures such as open-heart surgery. The tube is inserted into the patient's chest between the ribs to restore negative intrapleural pressure inside the chest wall; negative pressure is necessary to maintain the inflation of the lungs. The chest tube is connected to a drainage system to release air or to collect fluid and blood from the surrounding area with a hemothorax. The chest tube system is connected to wall suction to create negative pressure within the chest wall.

Pneumothorax is the result of air accumulating in the space between the lung and chest wall; a pneumothorax may occur spontaneously or may be the result of an injury to the patient's chest. Hemothorax is the accumulation of blood in the space between the lung and the chest wall; it may occur due to a blunt or penetrating traumatic injury. The occurrence of either a pneumothorax or hemothorax can result in a life-threatening emergency. If unrecognized and untreated, a tension pneumothorax may occur and result in cardiac arrest and patient death.

Complications may occur upon insertion of the chest tube; inexperienced resident doctors and even doctors with over a decade of clinical experience have encountered challenges or made mistakes inserting chest tubes. Tenured physicians are less likely to experience complications but may have an attitude of overconfidence contributing to mistakes if they are not vigilant during this procedure.

The multiple documented complications and adverse events caused by chest tube insertion include injury to the lung (55%), thoracic vascular injury (21%) liver injury (10%), spleen injury (4%) and damage to the intercostal blood vessels and nerves (Kamio et al., 2021). Unfortunately, "wrong side" chest tube insertions have been found to occur; placing the chest tube in the healthy side of the chest instead of the injured lung space is classified as a "never event" by the National Quality Forum and should *never* occur.

Appropriate nursing care following chest tube insertion is vital; the chest tube system must function properly to ensure the patient does not experience respiratory compromise. Patients must be monitored carefully for excessive bleeding, intercostal nerve and/or blood vessel damage, potential injury to vital organs after chest tube insertion, and infection. The amount and color of drainage in the collecting device is important to monitor; any excessive drainage or bright red blood can indicate the patient may be actively bleeding. The oscillation of fluid in the tubing is important to assess as it indicates a patent chest tube. The positioning of the tubing leading from the chest to the collecting device should be assessed; if it is kinked or coiled under the patient, pressure may build up in the chest wall and become a life-threatening emergency if untreated.

The tissue surrounding the chest tube insertion site should be softly palpated to assess for any subcutaneous air; this may indicate an "air leak" and should be monitored closely. The dressing over the insertion site should be changed daily. The skin around the tube should be assessed for signs of infection such as any redness, inflammation, or drainage around the insertion site. The nurse should assess the patient's laboratory results to check for an elevated white blood cell count or note an elevation in the patient's temperature as this may indicate a potential infection.

It is essential that the patient's vital signs are monitored closely, especially respiratory rate and oxygen saturation. Breath sounds should be auscultated at a minimum of every four hours and more frequently if the patient shows any signs of respiratory distress. The patient should be encouraged to cough and deep breathe at least every hour to encourage the inflation of the alveoli—the small air sacs in the lung where oxygen and carbon dioxide are exchanged. A collapse of the alveoli (due to shallow breathing) allows fluid to collect in this area and may lead to pneumonia. The physician will write the order for the patient's desired activity level. Unless contraindicated, the patient should be encouraged to sit up in the chair and to walk in the hallways; this activity encourages alveoli expansion contributing to pulmonary health.

It was found approximately half of nurses did not know how to care for a patient with a chest tube, with almost 58% stating they did not have prior training. Almost 35% of nurses said they did not utilize any resources to increase their knowledge in caring for a patient with a chest tube; they believed their current knowledge was sufficient. Over 36% of nurses stated they researched information about chest tubes on the internet using search engines rather than science-based databases. Information found on the internet can be inaccurate or invalid, leading to misinformation in caring for critical patients (Seyma et al., 2021). These statistics are scary; your nurse needs your help.

This information should empower you as a family member or loved one to advocate for safe and quality care. Ask questions and make sure the healthcare team understand you care and want to work together. You can alert the nurses if you observe something that concerns you or you don't understand.

A Femoral Sheath Fatality

After undergoing a scheduled percutaneous coronary intervention to visualize the coronary arteries with fluoroscopy, Mr. Smith was taken to the medical ward for observation and cared for. The hospital had recently converted several medical beds to monitored beds to provide specialized care for patients after cardiac procedures were performed. Mr. Smith was transferred from the cardiac catheterization laboratory to this nursing unit for further care and observation. He had the femoral artery sheath used for the procedure still in the femoral artery in his groin. The nurse caring for him removed the sheath as was ordered by the physician post-procedure. This nurse had inadequate training for this procedure and limited experience caring for these patients; she did not realize or anticipate the potential complications of removing arterial sheaths.

The nurse became busy with another patient she was caring for and neglected to assess Mr. Smith every 15 minutes as required by protocol. An hour later the patient was found unresponsive in a puddle of blood. A Code Blue was called, and Mr. Smith was transferred to the intensive care unit. Mr. Smith died several hours later; he had lost too much blood and could not be saved. This tragic loss of Mr. Smith's life could have been prevented with proper training, monitoring, and timely interventions.

The arteries are the high-pressure part of the vascular system; punctures in an artery (from a sheath placement) take longer for a "seal" to form by the internal clotting system. Direct manual pressure must be held on an arterial puncture site for a minimum of 5–10 minutes to ensure hemostasis; close monitoring ensures the puncture site has "sealed" enough to prevent rapid bleeding from the site. Frequent monitoring must be performed as there is a risk of bleeding if the patient coughs or moves enough to break the fragile seal.

As these situations can be catastrophic, Hildy Schell-Chaple, RN, PhD, of UCSF discusses the risks of bleeding events associated with femoral vascular access sheaths. Education and focused training must be expected and given to nurses caring for patients after interventional cardiac diagnostic procedures. The author highlights how applying a system's approach to practice changes can optimize safety and performance improvement outcomes (https://psent.ahrq.gov/webmm-case-studies).

KEY TAKEAWAYS

- In 2018, more than half of feeding tube placements were incorrect and were serious events.

- Incorrect feeding tube placements can cause serious harm or death.
- Chest x-ray is the definitive confirmation of correct feeding tube, nasogastric tube, and chest tube placements.
- A patient with a feeding tube needs the head of the bed elevated at least 30 degrees to avoid aspiration.
- A study in 2011 cited misplaced nasogastric tubes contributed to 21 deaths and 79 cases of harm.
- Failed intubations occur in over 20% of pre-hospital attempts outside of the hospital.
- Misplaced endotracheal tubes may contribute to death if unrecognized and uncorrected.
- Half of nurses do not know how to care for a patient with a chest tube.
- Patients with femoral sheaths must be monitored by trained nursing staff to prevent patient harm or death.

CHAPTER 17

CLINICAL DEVICE ALARMS

Why Would Anyone Silence a Patient Alarm?

In February 2013, 17-year-old Mariah Edwards was admitted to an outpatient surgical center to have her tonsils removed, a routine procedure performed by physicians thousands of times every year. The surgery went well; there were no complications experienced during the surgery. While in the post-surgery recovery room, Mariah was given a dose of Fentanyl for her pain, a potent opioid analgesic. Mariah's respiratory rate slowed significantly after receiving the Fentanyl; she was monitored electronically in the recovery room, but the alarms did not ring when her oxygen saturation fell into the critical zone. The nurse was busy caring for another patient at the time and did not notice Mariah's physiological deterioration.

Unobserved, Mariah's respiratory rate decreased until she was no longer breathing, resulting in cardiac arrest and her death. Mariah could not be resuscitated; her brain had been deprived of oxygen for too long. During the lawsuit, a nurse admitted the monitor alarms had been muted or silenced. These alarms are meant to alert healthcare staff to patient changes requiring urgent attention. The lawsuit settled for $6 million; no amount of money is worth the life of a daughter, family member, and friend.

The U.S. Food and Drug Administration cites a report indicating there were 566 alarm-related deaths between 2005 and 2008 (Jones, K., 2014). Advances in technology over the past few decades have provided the healthcare industry with over 40 medical devices developed and intended to improve patient care. Many of these commonly used medical devices today have built-in alarms to alert healthcare providers when patients need urgent action to keep them safe. Both bedside and remote monitors can measure vital signs, heart rhythms (ECG), oxygen saturation, and carbon dioxide levels. Ventilators to assist a patient's breathing are utilized when a patient is given general anesthesia, sedating medications and/or paralyzing medications necessary to perform a surgery or procedure. Intravenous pumps to regulate the flow rate of fluids and medications assist the accuracy needed to ensure the correct amount is delivered to the patient.

Clinical device alarms are designed to alert the medical staff to changes in the patients' physiological condition that may require attention or an intervention to prevent harm. They may also alarm if the device isn't functioning correctly and will need to be taken out of service (Lewandowska et al., 2020). Some clinical devices have built-in safety measures such as alarm parameters which can be customized to individual patients' needs. IV pumps can be programmed to deliver medications at a set rate; the pump will alarm if the flow of fluid is too slow or stops. Bed alarms can be added on the mattress of a patient who is at risk for falling or is confused; the alarm will signal when a patient is getting out of bed and alert the nurse to check on the patient.

Medical personnel need to be appropriately trained to use the equipment utilized in monitoring and caring for patients. It is essential that clinical devices are set up with clinical alarm parameters relevant to the patient's situation and needs. Alarms on clinical devices are meant to be lifesaving, but can compromise the safety of the patient if they are not promptly addressed or if misused. The very purpose of clinical monitors with alarms is to alert clinicians that a patient needs their urgent attention; they should *never* be in silent mode. The only time an alarm should be temporarily silenced is after the patient has been assessed. All healthcare facilities should have clinical device alarm policies to prevent disastrous patient outcomes.

Medical device companies recommend maintenance schedules, calibrations, and regular inspections to ensure devices function properly. The maintenance departments in healthcare facilities will typically manage the annual inspections of medical devices. Medical equipment can malfunction at times and require troubleshooting of the issue; it is vital that these devices are taken out of service until they can be repaired. A clinical device malfunction, a failure of a device, or delay or failure of a critical alarm can jeopardize patient safety.

Alarm Fatigue

Clinical alarm hazards have been one of the ECRI's (Emergency Care Research Institute) Top 10 Health Technology Hazards every year since the list's inception in 2007. "From 2009 and 2012, patient deaths were associated with 80 of the 98 alarm-related sentinel events voluntarily reported to the Joint Commission" (Ruppel et al., 2018). Medical staff can become overwhelmed, distracted, and desensitized to the noise of multiple or frequent alarms from medical devices.

The Joint Commission has estimated that 85–99% of clinical alarms do not require medical attention, and therefore, most nurses may disregard the alarms as meaningless. Nurses may become "numb" to the sound of repeated alarms; this is a survival mechanism and is not even a conscious decision. By "tuning out" the sound of frequent alarms, the healthcare provider may ignore a life-threatening alarm and compromise patient safety.

Alarm fatigue occurs more frequently in areas of the hospital where multiple monitors and medical devices with alarms are needed in caring for ill and critically ill patients. This cacophony of noise can create distractions and a feeling of "sensory overload"; it can be overwhelming and lead to a desensitization to the sound of a ringing alarm. ICU nurses have reported the continuous noise from the many alarms in caring for critical patients is burdensome and leads to a distrust that alarms are meaningful. In the ICU, studies found 85–99% of alarms were found to be insignificant; each patient's monitor was found to generate between 150–400 alarms per day, leading to desensitization (Lewandowska et al., 2020).

In January 2014, the Joint Commission added a new National Patient Safety Goal to target this growing syndrome of alarm fatigue (Wong, 2014). An alarm that is perceived as "false positive" may delay the nurse's response to check the patient's status (Graham, 2010). Fatigue is the lack of energy to react both psychologically and physiologically and may lead to an inadequate or delayed response to an alarm. Prolonged exposure to constant noise, such as in the ICU, can lead to a feeling of stress, irritation, or fear and result in decreased collaboration with other healthcare workers (Lewondowska et al., 2020).

Managing the noise levels in the hospital unit can be challenging. Adjusting the alarm parameters on any medical device to adjust alarm limits should follow institutional policy and should be done with caution. The healthcare provider may decide to adjust an alarm range of high or low levels due to the frequency of a "false-positive" situation occurring. For example, a patient's activity, such as brushing their teeth or frequently moving around in their bed, may be detected by the monitor as a rapid heart rate and may set off a false-positive alarm. Safe healthcare practice necessitates always checking and assessing the patient to ensure they are stable.

A high-pressure alarm on a ventilator may be "set off" and ring when the patient coughs; this is a common occurrence, especially when secretions are suctioned through the endotracheal (breathing) tube. A high-pressure alarm can also be caused by a bronchospasm, an obstruction in the endotracheal tube, or fluid pooling in the circuit. The alarm may be adjusted to be less sensitive to decrease the frequency of the alarm when the cause has been determined. Caution must always be used when adjusting alarm sensitivity. The healthcare provider must assess and determine the cause of the alarm to ensure the patient is stable and does not need intervention.

Clinical alarms are creating "a riot of disturbances for patients trying to heal and get some rest," according to a November 24, 2019, article in *The Washington Post*. The number of devices that generate alarms has grown from 10 to nearly 40 in the past 30 years, states the ECRI Institute senior project engineer Priyanka Shah. The sheer number of alarms is leading to a "cry wolf phenomenon," the author says, with overwhelmed providers ignoring alarms they think are meaningless. The Joint Commission now requires hospitals to use formal processes to tackle alarm safety, but no national data is available on progress in reducing unnecessary or false alarms (https://www.ecri.org/components/HRCAlerts/Pages/HRCAlerts112719_Ventilator.aspx).

Despite considerable recent improvements in alarm technology, further advancements are needed to improve the accuracy of alarms to be clinically relevant to detect physiological patient changes (Ruppel et al., 2018). The healthcare team needs accurate and sensitive alarms to signal when a patient may be in acute distress or needs immediate attention to improve patient safety. The ability to better discern between significant and insignificant alarms is necessary to decrease the frequency of "false" alarms and significantly reduce alarm fatigue.

KEY TAKEAWAYS

- 566 clinical device alarm-related deaths between 2005 and 2008.

- Clinical device alarms are designed to save patients' lives.
- Silencing monitor alarms contributes to patient harm and death.
- Utilization of multiple devices with alarms desensitizes staff to meaningful alerts.
- 85–99% of alarms are false or clinically insignificant; healthcare staff is ignoring alarms.
- Over a three-year period, 80 of the 98 sentinel events were alarm related.
- Alarm fatigue leads to desensitization of alarm "noise," resulting in healthcare professionals missing significant alarms and risking patient safety.

CHAPTER 18

PATIENT OBSERVATION
Scrutiny and Surveillance Required

Gabby was a healthy and vibrant five-year-old who tragically lost her life due to multiple failures of the healthcare system; her death was 100% preventable. This account is given by her loving father as he shared it with The Patient Safety Movement; he grieves every day for the loss of his daughter.

On May 1, Gabby became ill and woke up with a high fever of 102.5°F. She complained of nausea, a headache, had no appetite, and drank very little fluids. Her parents brought her to the pediatrician, where her throat swab for strep was negative; it was assumed she had a virus. Her fever continued for the next several days and then she broke out in a red-spotted rash all over her body. Her parents were quite concerned when her fever reached 105°F and took her to the Emergency Department (ED). The physician briefly examined her and stated her throat was red and swollen; he diagnosed Gabby with tonsillitis and stated the rash was from the fever. She was given an antibiotic and medication to bring down her fever and was discharged home.

For several more days, Gabby's fever remained between 103°F

and 104°F; she was tired, lethargic, and complained of abdominal and leg pain. Her parents took her to the pediatrician, who told them to stop the oral antibiotics because "this isn't tonsillitis" and "her fever should go down in the next day or two." Gabby was now getting agitated and off balance when she tried to walk; she was only taking sips of water so wasn't going to the bathroom.

On May 5, Gabby's fever reached 105°F, her parents were very worried and rushed her to the Emergency Department. The physician looked her over and didn't seem overly concerned; he ordered lab work and agreed to give her IV fluids at the urging of her parents. Her heart rate was elevated, her blood pressure was low, and she hadn't urinated in over 23 hours. At shift change, the new physician didn't come in to see Gabby for over six hours. Gabby finally did urinate just a little bit; her urine was reported to the physician to be dark in color. Her parents were told she was fine, even after the third inquiry of concern by Gabby's father. Dark urine and infrequent urine are signs of severe dehydration; this is especially concerning as she had been given IV fluids. When her parents inquired about the lab results, the physician told them the lab work "was all good" and he was discharging her home. Gabby was very tired and weak; she had to be carried out to the car.

On May 7, Gabby's condition had not improved; her father called the pediatrician's office and asked the nurse if they received copies of the lab work from the hospital. The nurse replied the doctor was reviewing the results now; he then heard the physician say, "Oh my God, her labs were awful! Tell them get her to the ED right away or call 911!" The lab test revealed 17 abnormal results and stated "Abnormal" on the top of the page; the results showed signs of sepsis and Systemic Inflammatory Response Syndrome (SIRS), a life-threatening situation.

Her new lab results were now even worse than before, yet she wasn't started on antibiotics for seven more hours. Later that evening, Gabby's vital signs were deteriorating; she experienced increasing respiratory distress and became unstable several hours later. The doctors inserted a breathing tube and transported her to another hospital by air ambulance. Her lungs filled with fluid, her body was swollen with third-spaced fluid due to the SIRS; she ultimately had swelling in her brain that cut off blood flow and oxygen.

Gabby did not survive this catastrophic week of medical errors and passed away on May 8th, a preventable and tragic death of a five-year-old girl who should have had her whole life in front of her. The healthcare team missed the diagnosis of Rocky Mountain Spotted Fever, and she was wrongly discharged from the ED. The diagnosis of sepsis and SIRS was missed because her lab work was dismissed or ignored by several healthcare providers. Gabby's very low urine output and deteriorating vital signs were red flags but ignored by the medical team until it was too late. Her parents end their account of this devastating experience by stating, "We shouldn't be visiting a cemetery every day."

As with our opening story of Lewis Blackman's tragedy in Chapter 1, there were multiple opportunities for any healthcare team member to step in and intervene. How did so many medical personnel miss asking appropriate questions and using clinical judgement to realize Gabby was very sick? We need to shine the spotlight on these multiple failures to recognize a deteriorating and unstable patient to learn from this family's experience. Gabby's parents did ask intelligent questions and brought valid concerns forward; why were they "dismissed" and placated with "all is good"? In hindsight, I'm sure they wished they had asked for a copy of the lab report, insisted on a second opinion, demanded to talk to the House Supervisor or Hospital Administrator on call, or anything that could have changed the trajectory of Gabby's life. They shared their heartbreaking experience to help other people going through a similar experience with their loved ones.

Twenty-eight percent of adverse events are related to areas of patient care (Levinson, 2010). There is a one in 300 chance that a patient will suffer harm in the healthcare system due to unsafe healthcare practices (Zaitoun et al., 2023). Competent nurses are essential contributors in cultivating and sustaining a safety culture in healthcare institutions. Nursing is a very complex job and requires high levels of responsibility as a key contributor to patient safety. Nursing competencies include foundational knowledge and key principles of patient care concepts such as physiology, pharmacology, communication, and safety. Critical thinking and clinical judgment are essential abilities and skill sets to synthesize patient data to prevent harm; nurses must be able to rapidly identify and respond appropriately to changes in a patient's condition (Zaitoun et al., 2023).

Nurses must know institutional policy and procedures to ensure best practices are followed to keep patients safe. Evidence-based research guides updates or revisions in best practices for healthcare delivery; organizations are responsible for updating policies and procedures based on scientific evidence. It is an expected standard that nurses utilize evidence-based practice (EBP) in guiding clinical practice (Cosme et al., 2018). Studies show that nurses' knowledge and skills vary based on educational level; nurses with graduate level education had the most knowledge of EBP principles followed by bachelor's prepared nurses, then associate degree prepared nurses. Advanced nursing education reflects a greater understanding of EBP as these skills are emphasized in graduate nursing programs and in Doctor of Nursing Practice (DNP) programs (Crawford et al., 2020).

As nurses spend 8 to 12 hours per day at or near a patient's bedside, they are ultimately accountable and responsible for the total care of patients. From my perspective as an experienced nurse and nurse educator, the following are particularly important considerations when planning and giving care to patients. If you are a patient or are a family member, this is essential information for you to be aware of as it may empower you to ask questions and to be the patient's advocate and keep them safe.

Fluid Volume

Management of patients' fluid balance is a crucial element of patient care in the acute care setting. The measurement of the patient's intake and output (I/O) is an expected part of the patient assessment and the nursing observation process. Exercising clinical judgment is the process of collecting relevant patient data; it is essential that the nurse utilize this process to anticipate potential patient problems and ensure good patient outcomes. It is very important to monitor I/O as an imbalance of body fluids may indicate a change in homeostasis and patient stability. Fluid overload or fluid deficit may be life-threatening if not observed and corrected with appropriate intervention.

Physicians may order I/O and daily weights to be measured for patients who may be at risk for complications if the body fluid volume becomes imbalanced. Thielen (2014) cited that the deaths of 8.5% of patients with fluid overload were due to a lack of monitoring and communication by the healthcare team. Daily weights are the most accurate method and considered the "gold standard" to measure changes in the patient's fluid volume status. Many hospital beds have integrated scales to weigh the patient when they are unable to stand. To obtain an accurate reading, it is important the patient is weighed with the same linens on the bed each time.

Some medical conditions, such as congestive heart failure (CHF) or kidney dysfunction, may result in an excess of fluid retained in the body, placing the patient at risk for complications. Patients with CHF are prone to fluid overload if the heart muscle is not strong enough to effectively pump all the blood out into the body. The blood can backflow from the heart back into the lungs, causing breathing difficulties. Excess fluid in the lungs prevents the gas exchange of oxygen and carbon dioxide in the alveoli and may lead to respiratory dysfunction. A patient experiencing kidney dysfunction may be placed on a strict fluid restriction; if the kidneys are not functioning optimally, fluid volume overload may occur.

In measuring fluid intake, any food that is liquid at room temperature such as jello, ice cream and popsicles must be counted in the intake measurement. Yes, patients can get very thirsty on a fluid restriction diet and can be very convincing when they attempt to get more to drink. I've found patients drinking out of the faucet in their hospital rooms because they were so thirsty. As a family member, nurses may need your support in helping the patient understand the reason the fluids are being restricted and ensuring they comply with the physician's order.

It is very important during and after surgery to monitor the patient's intake and output. During surgery, body fluid balance may shift; the potential loss of blood and other body fluids, or the infusion of IV fluids and/or blood products may cause a fluid imbalance. Remember from Chapter 1 when Lewis Blackman had low urine output in the recovery room? The pain medication he was given was contraindicated in low urine output states and contributed to his poor outcome and death. Any significant blood loss and fluid loss may need to be replaced with intravenous fluids to prevent dehydration and body fluid volume deficit.

Laboratory Examinations

It is essential to measure the patient's blood levels of various levels of elements found normally in the human body; it is one of the most frequently utilized diagnostic tools in assessing a patient's health. The maintenance of "normal" levels of electrolytes and blood components is essential for optimal physiological function and patient health. Electrolyte levels must be maintained within an identified narrow range for normal and optimal physiological function. For example, potassium is an essential electrolyte for cardiac function; if it is too high or too low, the patient may suffer dysrhythmias or cardiac arrest.

When you have a diagnostic test taken, find out when the

results are expected to come back; do not assume that no news is good news. Laboratory tests can vary in the time it takes to receive results. Common and simple tests such as complete blood counts or electrolyte values usually can be processed quickly; results are usually ready in a few minutes to a few hours. Other examinations such as a blood culture or a tissue biopsy may take several days to process in the laboratory.

The diagnostic process requires a physician to see the test result, interpret it correctly, and develop a plan of care to treat the patient. Some lab tests may need to be repeated if significantly abnormal or after an intervention is implemented to correct the abnormality. Some abnormal labs will not need immediate intervention or treatment and may need to be monitored to track the trending of the lab value.

The following are a few examples of commonly ordered lab tests:

- **Glucose**—imbalance can cause irritability, seizures, coma, cardiac irregularity, and brain impairment
- **Sodium**—regulates nerves, muscles, and body fluid composition; imbalance can cause seizures, coma, and death
- **Potassium**—essential for smooth muscle contraction; imbalance can cause cardiac dysrhythmias, cardiac arrest, and death
- **Calcium**—essential for muscle contraction, regulating normal heart rhythms and blood clotting
- **Hemoglobin**—carries oxygen, removes carbon dioxide, evaluates anemia and blood loss
- **White Blood Cell count**—evaluates bacterial or viral infection, can indicate bone marrow dysfunction
- **Platelets**—essential for normal clotting of blood

Unfortunately, a significant number of abnormal test results are not reported to the physician or not acted on in a timely

manner. Failure to report abnormal lab values or lack of appropriate action may lead to significant patient harm. Failure to follow
up on critical tests may result in the delay of a timely diagnosis
or interventions to improve the patient's outcome. For example,
some diuretic medications will increase the excretion of potassium; if the patient's potassium levels are low, the medication
may cause a further loss of potassium. As potassium is essential
for cardiac function, the patient may be at risk for cardiac dysrhythmias including cardiac arrest.

In a study measuring missed diagnoses in the emergency
department, 79 of the 122 legal claims cite patient harm resulting from missed laboratory or radiological test results (Callen et
al., 2011). This "miss" may result in potential patient harm, poor
patient outcomes, and may contribute to patient deaths. Many
healthcare systems allow the patient to view the results of diagnostic tests via a patient portal after the physician has released
them. Remember, access to your own medical record is one of
your patient "rights."

Always request access to your personnel health information
on your patient portal; you may see critical values before you hear
from your physician. The data you see should reflect the normal
ranges of each specific laboratory examination and your results.
It is important to understand the implications of any abnormal
results you may see; your physician should discuss the results of
your tests and if you should expect any impact to your health.
For example, if the patient's platelet count is low (normal range
is between 150,000 and 450,000 platelets per microliter of blood),
patients are at risk for bleeding and need to be observed for bruising, bleeding gums, and blood in the urine or stool.

Learn as much as you can about your health condition and
treatments. Remember, you should be an active participant in
your own healthcare. Ask your healthcare providers and nurses
questions and try to educate yourself as much as you can by utilizing reliable sources. You can find various treatment options

that are based on the latest scientific research and evidence at this website: https://www.effectivehealthcare.ahrq.gov.

Find out if the treatment recommended for you or your loved one is based on the latest scientific evidence.

Patient Falls

Bill A. was suffering from a hip injury which required surgery to restore his mobility and minimize his pain. Several days later, he was successfully recovering from the surgery when the nurse helped him walk to the bathroom. She left him alone in the bathroom while she went to attend to another patient. Bill was tired and wanted to get back to bed; he knew he was weak but thought he would be able to get to his bed unassisted. Unfortunately, he lost his balance and fell, hitting his head and injuring his neck. The doctors ordered traction to keep Bill's neck in alignment with his body to promote healing and prevent further injury.

The neck traction allows only minimal activity and required Bill to lie on his back for long periods of time. It required two to three nurses to help him move around and change positions. Bill's decreased physical activity and difficulty taking deep breaths post-operatively led to the development of pneumonia. Bill was placed on a ventilator to help him breathe; his condition was critical and required close observation in the intensive care unit (ICU). The increased length of stay contributed to Bill acquiring methicillin-resistant *Staphylococcus aureus* (MRSA) while in the ICU; this was followed with another infection, *clostridium difficile* (c. diff). Devastatingly, Bill lost his life after the multiple health challenges he encountered after falling after his hip surgery. His battle with two hospital-acquired infections was too much for his body to recover from.

A patient fall is defined as an unplanned descent to the floor with or without injury to the patient. Falls resulting in a serious injury are consistently ranked in the Top 10 Sentinel Events reported to the Joint Commission. Each year, somewhere between 700,000 and 1,000,000 people in the United States suffer a fall in the hospital (AHRQ). In another study, the occurrence of patient falls estimates 11 patient falls per 1,000 patient days, increasing the cost of the hospital stay by over $30K per event and increasing the length of stay up to 45 days (Watson et al., 2019). Unfortunately, research shows that the rate of patient falls incurring significant injuries has increased over 17% since the COVID-19 pandemic in 2020 (Fleisher et al., 2022).

Higher rates of falls have been documented in the elderly population; older patients may be confused in the unfamiliar setting of the hospital, leading to risk of accidental falls. The aging process may contribute to less muscle mass, leaving this population weaker and more vulnerable to frailty and falls. All age ranges of patients may be at risk for falls due to effects of medications such as sedatives and pain medication; caution and close observation should be implemented with these high-risk patients. Fall prevention involves managing a patient's underlying fall risk factors; medical conditions, diagnostic, and surgical procedures can leave patients vulnerable to falls. Close observation should be considered when planning care for these patients to prevent the incidence of falls and improve outcomes.

Serious negative outcomes may occur from patient fall events and include the inability to return home, increased potential to fall again, physical injury, and even death. A fall may result in fractures, lacerations, or internal bleeding, contributing to increased health care costs, further patient complications, and poor outcomes. Research shows that close to one-third of falls can be prevented. As of 2008, the Centers for Medicare and Medicaid Services (CMS) does not reimburse hospitals for certain types of traumatic injuries that occur while a patient is in the hospital.

Preventing patient falls is a focus and priority for many healthcare organizations. Several practices have been shown to reduce the occurrence of falls, but these practices are not used systematically in all hospitals. Tracking patient falls and identifying contributing factors may help organizations decrease the incidence of these adverse events (Watson et al., 2019).

Various fall prevention programs and initiatives have been implemented to decrease patient falls; unfortunately, the statistics demonstrate a low success rate. A strategy implemented at one healthcare system placed yellow identification bands on patients to identify them as a high risk for falls to hospital staff. Designated signs placed on the patient's door indicate the patient is at high risk for falls; one facility used the picture of a tree on its side to preserve patient confidentiality. Assessing the patient environment is essential to identify potential safety hazards and prevent an accident. Hospital personnel need to treat the problem that prompted the patient's admission, keep the patient safe, and help the patient maintain or recover physical and mental function (https://www.ahrq.gov/patient-safety/settings/hospital/fall-prevention/toolkit/index.html#Problem).

Pressure Ulcers

Each year, more than 2.5 million people in the United States develop pressure ulcers; it is the third most costly disease. Pressure ulcers are a worldwide preventable health care issue contributing to over 60,000 deaths each year (Borojeny et al., 2020). These skin lesions bring pain, associated risk for serious infection, and increased health care utilization. Pressure ulcers are associated with longer hospital stays and increased morbidity and mortality (Borojeny et al., 2020).

Pressure ulcers are a healthcare priority and rank near the top of preventable occurrences in hospitals and long-term care facilities, affecting hundreds of thousands of patients every year. Pressure ulcers, decubitus ulcers, or "bed sores" develop when there is an interference of the blood flow caused by pressure. If the pressure is unrelieved, it may result in injury to the skin and underlying tissue and expose the patient to potential bacterial infections. The most common areas affected by pressure and lack of blood flow are along bony prominences such as the tailbone, heels, shoulders, ears, the back of the head, hips, and elbows.

The skin is the largest organ of the human body and has important protective functions. The skin:

- Protects the body from mechanical, thermal, or chemical injury.
- Is a protective barrier to prevent bacteria from entering and invading the body.
- Helps regulate body temperature.
- Is a sensory organ for pressure, touch, pain, cold and heat.

Body fluid is retained by the skin and prevents external fluid from being absorbed. The skin is made up of two primary layers, the epidermis and the dermis, with a third layer of subcutaneous tissue made up of fat cells for more protection. A break in the skin integrity may expose the patient to multiple complications; it is an essential component of patient safety to ensure skin integrity is maintained.

Identifying high-risk patients is the first step in preventing the development of pressure injuries that can erode the skin, causing infection, pain, and reduced quality of life for the patient. Patients at high risk of pressure injuries may have mobility limitations or decreased activity, an altered mental status, lower mental awareness, or decreased sensory perception. Other risk factors for pressure ulcers include obesity, increased age, dehydration, excess fluid volume, and malnutrition.

Prevention of pressure ulcers is a high priority for patients identified as high risk. Minimizing the pressure on any area of the body by turning and repositioning the patient at least every two hours is essential. If the patient doesn't or can't turn themselves, staff or family members must do this for them. Skin breakdown can occur very quickly; skin inspection should be performed frequently on all patients who are at risk. Friction and shearing of the skin can occur if the patient is moved improperly;

it may cause serious injuries and lead to infection and pain for the patient. It is important the staff or caregivers use caution when moving a patient to keep the skin intact to prevent injury.

Healthcare facilities may utilize pressure-reducing beds or mattresses and foam pads to decrease pressure injuries. Heavy workloads and short staffing are pervasive across healthcare environments resulting in infrequent skin assessments and prevention strategies for high-risk patients. Educating family caregivers in the early stages of skin changes and engaging them in pressure injury prevention is an effective strategy to minimize patient injury (Taylor et al., 2021).

KEY TAKEAWAYS

- 28% of adverse events are related to areas of patient care.
- One in 300 chances a patient will suffer harm in the healthcare system due to unsafe practices.
- The deaths of 8.5% of patients with fluid overload were due to a lack of monitoring and communication by the healthcare team.
- Laboratory results are crucial information—ask to see the results. Don't assume "all is good."
- 79 of 122 legal claims cite patient harm resulting from missed laboratory or radiological test results.
- Between 700,000 and 1,000,000 patients in the U.S. suffer a fall in the hospital.
- One-third of patient falls can be prevented.
- Pressure ulcers impact 2.5 million people in the U.S. and cause 60,000 deaths worldwide.

CHAPTER 19

SURGERY, PROCEDURES, AND BLOOD TRANSFUSIONS

Things You Must Know to Remain Safe

Ms. Young, a 72-year-old female was admitted to the hospital to undergo a minor procedure for postmenopausal bleeding. She experienced more bleeding than was expected and low blood pressure during surgery. Her laboratory results showed low hemoglobin and hematocrit levels; she was transfused with two units of packed red blood cells. The next morning, the patient complained of severe abdominal pain and nausea. By the afternoon, her heart rate had elevated to 145 beats per minute and her EKG showed she was in an atrial fibrillation rhythm. The cardiologist prescribed a blood thinner (to prevent blood clots that can occur with this heart rhythm); her hemoglobin level was still low after the blood transfusion.

The patient continued to have nausea and abdominal pain; by evening she had an episode of bloody vomitus. Her laboratory values were not re-checked; her blood thinner medication was continued. The following morning, the patient's hemoglobin had dropped to a critical level of 5.8 g/Dl. Ms. Young was now confused and exhibiting severe signs of shock. Her vital signs had deteriorated drastically; her blood pressure had dropped to reflect severe hypotension of 75/45 mm Hg and her heart rate elevated to 130 beats per minute. Unfortunately, the patient went into cardiac arrest and could not be resuscitated. Her death was attributed to ischemia in her bowel complicated by gastrointestinal bleeding. The healthcare team missed many signs of patient deterioration. "Perioperative deaths are often the culmination of a cascade of discrete clinical events; there is no such thing as a minor procedure in surgery" (Ghaferi, 2017).

Informed Consent

Veracity (truth telling) is the moral and ethical principle defining the patient's right to have a clear understanding of information regarding their health and plan of care (Bonney, 2014). "Informed Consent" is the process that includes the structured conversation between physician and patient to communicate recommended treatments, procedures, or surgeries. It is required by law and necessitates the consent of the patient or guardian to agree to undergo a procedure or surgery. The patient must be at least 18 years of age, mentally competent, and must not have been given any mind-altering medications prior to signing the Informed Consent document. Signing the Informed Consent document indicates the patient has been involved in the decision-making process for their care. If the patient has second thoughts and changes their mind, the Informed Consent can be withdrawn at any time prior to the surgery procedure.

The healthcare provider must give the patient the information about the proposed procedure or surgery in an easy-to-understand manner. The Informed Consent for the proposed procedure or surgery must include:

- the risks and benefits of the procedure
- the potential consequences of opting out of the procedure

- the name of the healthcare provider who will perform the procedure

When a patient is told by their healthcare provider that a surgery, procedure, or test is necessary, it is important for the patient to understand why a test or treatment is needed. It is required that the intended outcome or benefit to your health is explained to you. There is a chance you may not really need the recommended treatment; it is *always* your option to get a second opinion. You can and should do your own research on your health condition and the test or procedure being recommended to you. When you are fully informed and understand your options and the consequences of having or not having the procedure, you need to determine if it is right for you.

The Surgical Setting

Of the various types of medical errors that occur, "surgical errors have the most direct and serious consequences, such as death or permanent injury. One in ten postoperative Medicare patients die from complications such as developing a pulmonary embolism/deep-vein thrombosis, pneumonia, sepsis, shock, cardiac arrest, or a GI hemorrhage (Verillo & Winters, 2018). The annual cost of medical errors "likely exceeds $17 billion, with 35% being surgery related" (Cohen et al., 2021). Approximately 14% of surgical patients in hospitals will experience at least one adverse event; these range from minor events to fatalities (Anderson et al., 2013). Factors contributing to peri-operative errors include overconfidence of the surgeon, distractions, mental fatigue, and focused attention on a single issue (Thiels et al., 2015).

Perioperative and intraoperative medical errors continue to occur at unacceptable rates, resulting in devastation for both patients and healthcare providers (Landers, 2015). It is challenging to understand the accurate number of adverse events that occur in the surgical suite; the highly litigious climate found in the healthcare environment contributes to the under-reporting of these adverse events. Surgeons are willing to report intraoperative adverse events, but systematically and significantly underreport them, especially if the event is considered lower severity (Peponis et al., 2018).

Research has demonstrated that although many intraoperative adverse events are of low severity, the injuries resulting from errors during surgery can be catastrophic. Thirty-five percent of documented *never events* occurred during major surgeries and include wrong procedure, 35%; wrong site/side, 30%; retained foreign object, 28%; and wrong implant, 7% (Thiels et al., 2015). Inadvertent injury to organs and vascular structures occurs too frequently during surgeries; injury to the bowel and vascular system are the most-cited structural injuries during surgery (Peponis et al., 2018).

Healthcare professionals trained to administer anesthesia during surgery can be either a medically trained doctor or a Certified Nurse Anesthetist. Delivering anesthesia requires the provider to have the ability to manage multiple tasks of acute patient management. Prioritization of vital signs regulation, airway and ventilator management for patients receiving general anesthetic agents, and ensuring patients stay asleep for the procedure are essential for optimal patient outcomes. Patients in critical condition pose a very complex and challenging situation requiring close surveillance and rapid interventions when necessary. Problems may occur during the administration of anesthesia during procedures or surgeries; this area of discipline requires a high-level of intense vigilance to keep patients safe. In their study, De Cassi et al. (2021) report that medication recording errors occurred at a rate as high as one in every eight administrations in the operative arena.

As discussed in Chapter 3, retained foreign bodies (RFB) after surgery are considered a *never event* that unfortunately still occurs many times per year. A forgotten surgical instrument, needles, surgical sponges or swabs left inside the patient's body can cause pain, infection, sepsis, and death. In a study from 2012 to 2020, 797 general surgical *never events* were reported, with 165 (46.5%) of the cases related to retained surgical swabs (Omar et al., 2021). Interventions implemented in many surgical suites include counting instruments and sponges, but research has shown that 77%–80% of presumably "correct counts" have resulted in RFB (Verma, 2021). Complications resulting from RFB may increase the length of stay and increase costs for these affected patients; some patients will need another surgery to remove the RFB, adding thousands of dollars to the cost of care.

Unfortunately, procedures performed on the wrong site, wrong side, the wrong patient, or the wrong procedure performed on a patient occur all too often. These types of medical errors are 100 percent preventable and are classified as *never events* as we discussed earlier. Surgical checklists now exist in many hospitals; utilization of surgical checklists in operating suites have been shown to decrease medical errors and even death (Harris et al., 2020).

Prior to surgery, it is expected that surgeons discuss the specific surgery with the patient, sign the Informed Consent, and sign their initials directly on the site of the body to be operated on. Because this type of error is usually obvious when it occurs, almost 90% of legal claims and lawsuits settle quickly and in favor of the patient. The liability is on the healthcare provider to perform his or her due diligence before beginning a procedure to ensure the correct surgery is performed.

Equipment failures or improper use of the medical equipment in the operating suite during the surgery may result in harm to the patient. Electrocautery equipment has been utilized during surgeries to minimize bleeding and help keep the surgical site visible to the surgeon. Many surgeons may not have formal training in the application of electrocautery equipment and may cause an intraoperative burn if recommended safety standards and caution are not utilized.

Post-operative Care

Lenore Alexander tragically lost her 11-year-old daughter, Leah, to a preventable medical error after a routine surgery. Leah was receiving Fentanyl, an opioid pain medication through an epidural catheter. Leah's father expressed his concern that he believed his daughter was way overmedicated; the resident physician replied that he would prescribe her some medicine for anxiety. Leah was given 2 mg of Ativan, a dose appropriate for a large man, not an 80-pound child.

Leah died several hours later with her mother asleep at her bedside. Leah was not on any electronic monitors, which could have detected a change in her vital signs and alerted someone that she was too sedated and in danger. The nurses or healthcare providers did not assess Leah frequently enough; they didn't notice when her breathing and her heart slowed to a stop. They didn't notice Leah's deterioration until it was too late; tragically, she could not be resuscitated.

Over 10% of post-operative patients develop serious complications within the first week, and 10.6% of post-operative patients were found to deteriorate and die. A single complication often leads to a second complication; multiple complications that can be life-threatening. The research showed that the most common post-operative complication is bleeding, followed by septic shock, pneumonia, respiratory failure, wound dehiscence, acute renal failure, cardiac arrest, and stroke (Ferraris et al., 2014).

Pain control is an important aspect of post-operative care and may assist in an optimal recovery. As we discussed in Chapter 15, the highest risk of administering opioid medications to a patient is potential respiratory depression. Patients receiving opioid therapy need to be assessed and monitored closely and frequently. The patient's respiratory rate per minute should be measured and counted at least every two hours and more frequently depending on the patient's status. Electronic monitoring devices can alert the nurse or healthcare provider to changes in vital signs and signal any potential patient deterioration.

Monitoring devices readily available in healthcare settings that perform procedures and surgeries should be utilized on all patients; these include oxygen saturation, heart rate, automatic blood pressure cuffs set on close intervals, and capnography monitors. Capnography monitors measure the value of exhaled carbon dioxide and are very sensitive to the changes in respiratory rate; they can alert the healthcare staff to patient decompensation much earlier than oxygen saturation monitors (SpO2). You can request and even demand that your loved one be monitored electronically at the very least; it is a standard of care and is expected procedure in the delivery of safe patient care.

The level of monitoring and patient care given after surgery may vary due to the complexity or specificity of the surgery as well as the patient's underlying level of health. The patient may be admitted to the intensive care unit or general care floor depending on the level of nursing care and observation needed. The patient may have surgical drains in place, dressings, various tubes, multiple intravenous solutions, pumps, and complex monitoring machines.

Pneumonia is the third most common post-operative complication; it may increase the patient's length of stay and cost up to $52K for additional hospital care (Caparelli et al., 2019). If the patient received general anesthesia during surgery, the incidence of pneumonia may be significantly increased. Post-operative pneumonia is a preventable complication that may occur several days after surgery if the alveoli (air sacs in the lungs) are not expanded sufficiently with air. The alveoli may fill with fluid, preventing gas exchange, if not inflated sufficiently by adequate respiratory effort by the patient.

The patient needs to take deep breaths, cough, and actively use the incentive spirometer (IS) every two hours while awake to expand the alveoli and optimize gas exchange. It is very important for the nurse and respiratory therapist to explain the importance of utilizing an "incentive spirometer" and demonstrate to the patient and family how to use it. Yes, it can cause operative site pain when the patient takes deep breaths and coughs, but the benefit is healthy lung function and the prevention of post-operative pneumonia.

Mobility is also very important after surgery. Years ago, healthcare providers thought keeping patients in bed for several days and limiting their activity was good for the patient and allowed them to heal; mobility was not encouraged or approved of. Several decades ago, patients having babies or undergoing open heart surgery were prescribed very limited activity; today, they're assisted to sitting up in the chair within a few short hours after surgery or childbirth. Research has demonstrated the benefit of getting the patient up and moving as soon as possible. Patients heal faster when activity is encouraged and supported; the oxygen and nutrients are circulated around the body when the patient is moving and active.

Venous Thromboembolism

Charles "Yogiraj" Bates experienced a brain injury from a fall that resulted in significant bleeding in his brain. He underwent surgery to evacuate the blood in his brain, as it was causing pressure inside his skull; he came through the surgery without any complications. Several days later, Charles started experiencing alarming symptoms including shortness of breath, chest pain, low oxygen levels, arm numbness, and lower leg pain. The healthcare team dismissed Charles's many concerning symptoms. His condition deteriorated and he suffered a grand mal seizure, he was transferred to the intensive care unit. By this time, his wife was very alarmed and stated, "we knew something was not right."

Charles had developed a venous thromboembolism after his surgery, causing the unexpected and dangerous symptoms he displayed and the subsequent seizure. Sadly, Charles did not survive these complications. Post-operative preventative measures could have avoided these complications and Charles's death; unfortunately, the healthcare team did not follow these measures.

After extensive review of her husband's medical records and inquiry with healthcare experts, Vonda Bates realized what had caused her husband's death. Charles "Yogiraj" Bates died from a preventable post-surgical complication. Regrettably, after multiple attempts to communicate and meet with the physicians and hospital administrators, the manager of the patient representative services told her, "Patients die in the hospital every day." How utterly tragic.

Acutely ill hospitalized patients are at risk for blood clots that may result in patient harm or death. Pulmonary embolism (PE) and deep vein thrombosis (DVT), collectively known as venous thromboembolism (VTE), represent a major public health problem that affects 350,000 to 600,000 Americans annually.

VTE has been identified to be among the most common preventable causes of hospital death (https://www.ahrq.gov/patient-safety/settings/hospital/vtguide/index.html). Estimates vary widely, but the overall annual prevalence of VTE may be increasing and can impact any patient who is immobile for extended lengths of time. VTEs are the most common preventable hospital complication; it is primarily a problem of sick or injured patients who are hospitalized or were recently hospitalized. Abboud et al. (2020) report that over 28,000 hospitalized patients die from VTE each year.

Certain procedures have been documented to have a high risk of VTE; these include abdominal or pelvic surgery for cancer, multiple major traumas, craniotomy and spinal surgery for malignant disease, and other spinal surgeries. Patients undergoing chest or esophagus surgeries are also at higher risk for VTE; most other surgical procedures requiring hospitalization fall into the moderate-risk category.

Evidence-based research demonstrates that the following interventions decrease the occurrence of VTE: encouraging patient mobility, the use of compression stockings, and utilizing a sequential compression device when the patient is on bedrest (Maynard, 2015). Patient activity and mobility are a simple and very effective intervention that both healthcare staff and families can engage in to prevent venous thromboembolism (VTE) postoperatively.

Anticoagulation medications are frequently administered to the patient postoperatively to prevent blood clots; a common anticoagulant medication is given subcutaneously using a very small needle to deliver the powerful medication right into the layer of fat under the skin. VTE prevention with anticoagulants is considered standard of care for major lower extremity surgeries.

Procedural Sedation

Sedative medications can be administered during medical procedures for patient comfort and amnesiac effects. Sedatives can be given during diagnostic procedures such as colonoscopies, and for therapeutic or painful procedures such as putting a dislocated joint or limb back in proper position. These procedures are usually performed in the emergency department, intensive care unit, or endoscopy suites where patients can be electronically monitored and closely observed.

The healthcare provider performing the procedure requiring sedation must be properly trained to do the procedure; they must possess the skill set "airway management" if the patient becomes unstable during the procedure. They must have healthcare team support such as a nurse and respiratory therapist to assist them if the patient requires airway support. "Joint Commission standards require practitioners to have a minimum skill set including the ability to manage a compromised airway and rescue patients who drift into deeper levels of sedation than anticipated" (Krauss & Green, 2008).

Sedative medications may cause a slowing of the patient's respiratory rate and can lead to decreased oxygen available for the brain and vital organs. During and after the procedure, close observation is mandatory to quickly identify any patient compromise and initiate early and rapid intervention if necessary. Respiratory failure or respiratory arrest may occur if the patient is unobserved, or appropriate interventions are not taken by the nurse or healthcare team. Sedated patients are at high risk for complications and must be monitored closely until the medication's sedative effects have worn off.

After the procedure, patients should not be given anything to drink or eat until they are fully awake and able to talk; this ensures that the airway's protective, laryngeal reflexes have returned. It is highly recommended these patients be electronically monitored; both oxygen saturation *and* capnography should be evaluated to ensure oxygen *and* ventilation are adequate. Appropriate monitoring equipment should be utilized; patient safety groups have long recognized and published the value of this lifesaving measure.

Blood Transfusions

Although it is rare, people can die from a blood transfusion reaction. In July 2019 at a prominent cancer hospital, a young woman died after receiving a blood transfusion. The investigators found the blood she was given had been contaminated with bacteria and believe that the blood transfusion protocol may not have been followed. Frequent monitoring of vital signs (temperature, blood pressure, respiratory rate, and pulse rate) and assessing the patient during the transfusion is the policy found in most healthcare facilities.

The investigation in this tragedy revealed that only 18 of the 36 patients receiving blood transfusions were properly monitored during the transfusion. "Of the over 17 million blood transfusions given in 2017, 37 patients died from a direct result of the transfusion, according to the Food and Drug Administration" (Hixenbaugh, 2019). Many of the nurses interviewed during this investigation stated they were unaware that the vital signs should have been checked (although the institution had a protocol outlining the procedure). Closely monitoring patients during a blood transfusion is a critical intervention and expectation of the registered nurse and healthcare staff; this is a core concept that is taught in nursing school curricula.

The administration of blood products (whole blood, packed red blood cells, plasma, or platelets) requires a physician's order. This procedure is not without risk; blood products should not be given unless clearly indicated by the patient's health condition. The physician must explain the risk versus benefit and necessity of the blood transfusion to the patient. The patient or the patient's guardian must sign an Informed Consent to give permission for the transfusion of any blood products.

A "type and crossmatch" laboratory test will be performed to identify the patient's blood type and tissue match to determine donor/recipient compatibility. The blood bank inventory process requires the matching blood product to be held in inventory for three days for the patient for whom it was ordered. If the patient does not need and receive the transfusion after three days, the blood product on hold is released for another patient to use if needed. If the patient needs a blood product transfusion after three days, another type and crossmatch will need to be obtained to secure the blood product ordered.

Receiving a transfusion of a blood product is not without risks, as we discussed in the case of the unfortunate young woman in 2019. Blood product transfusion reactions can be harmful and even fatal. Potential risks of receiving blood products are:

- Donor and recipient blood type incompatibility. This error is classified as a *"never event"* as it results from human error and is 100% preventable.
- Bacteria or viruses could contaminate blood product.
- Breathing problems may occur if the patient becomes

"fluid overloaded" due to the transfusion. This may occur in patients with compromised cardiac function.
- Allergic reaction to the blood product. This is the most common but unpredictable adverse event in transfusion risks.

Policy and procedures have been written and adopted in healthcare settings to minimize the risk of an adverse event; many of these include a checklist to ensure all steps in the transfusion process are followed accurately. The role of the nurse is to closely monitor the patient for adverse reactions during the transfusion to prevent patient harm or even death. Essential steps in the transfusion process include:

- Informed Consent is signed (unless emergent, life-threatening condition).
- Obtain pre-transfusion vital signs.
- Ensure the patient's intravenous site is patent and large enough to accommodate the blood product (a minimum of a 20-gauge angiocath, 18-gauge is preferred).
- Set up the filtered blood tubing with normal saline.
- Provide correct identification of the patient (two nurses required).
- Cross-check the blood component barcode number with the patient's blood band (two nurses required).
- Frequently monitor the patient's vital signs (every 15 minutes after the start of the transfusion).
- Monitor the patient's status for shortness of breath or difficulty breathing, complaints of back or abdominal pain, itching, hives or feeling "like my throat is closing off."
- STOP the blood transfusion immediately if the patient complains or has symptoms indicating a transfusion reaction or if the patient becomes unstable.
- Blood components expire after four hours out of the

refrigerator and must be infused into the patient within the four-hour period to prevent bacterial growth.

Healthcare research demonstrates the positive impact on patient safety and improved outcomes when patients and their families take an active role in their safety. Unfortunately, there has not been enough support and encouragement from health-care systems to promote this partnership. Harris et al., 2020) cite the clear impact on patient outcomes when a multidisciplinary program was implemented; peri-operative complications were reduced by 50% and mortality rates decreased by 42%.

KEY TAKEAWAYS

- 35% of *never events* occurred during major surgeries: wrong procedure, 35%; wrong site/side, 30%; retained foreign object 28%.
- Over 10% of post-operative patients develop serious complications within the first week.
- Over 28,000 hospitalized patients die from Venous Thromboembolism (VTE) each year.
- VTE is among the most common preventable causes of hospital death.
- Interventions prevent VITE and save lives—activity, compression stockings, and anticoagulant medications.
- Patients receiving sedation for procedures are at high risk for respiratory and central nervous system depression.
- Blood transfusion reactions can harm or kill a patient.
- Close patient monitoring is required during blood transfusions.
- Patient involvement in their own safety decreased complications by 50% and mortality by 42%.

CONCLUSION

Today, unfortunately, patient safety still does not exist to the extent it is needed and deserved. Patients continue to die unnecessarily despite technology and advances in medical discipline and practices (Bates et al., 2023). Healthcare leaders and practitioners must prioritize patient safety to support practices and accountability to impact outcomes we so desperately need. "To achieve the highest level of patient safety and to be able to reduce medical error and adverse events, one needs to recognize patient safety as a health priority in health sector policies and programs, collaborate with other member states along with the improvement of national policies, programs, guidelines, strategies and tools" (Ahsani-Estahbanati et al., 2022).

In November 2022, Health and Human Services (HHS)

Secretary Xavier Becerra startled a recent meeting of senior health system leaders by declaring in his opening remarks: "We're losing pretty much an airline full of Americans every day to medical error, but we don't think about it. The worst part about it is that it's avoidable." This appears to have signaled a renewed commitment by Health and Human Services (HHS) to preventing patient harm as it launched an "Action Alliance to Advance Patient Safety." The department's fiscal 2022–2026 strategic plan estimated the death toll at roughly 550 patients daily. The Alliance aims to recruit the nation's largest health systems as participants (*Forbes* magazine).

Many health system leaders emphasized the safety impact of workforce woes, financial stress, and the burden of often confusing regulations; all these challenges have been exacerbated by the recent COVID-19 pandemic. Patient safety advocates, however, sounded a very different tone. "You are focused on financial issues, on staffing," said Helen Haskell of Consumers Advancing Patient Safety. "But a failure to be transparent with patients [when harm occurs] is a key reason patient safety has not advanced." (Remember from Chapter 1, Helen Haskell is Lewis Blackman's mother.)

"For the past twenty years there has been a focus on the private-public partnership," said Armando Nahum, of Patients for Patient Safety (U.S.). "While we have seen some organizations step up to the plate, our system has not. Our federal government has not enforced its own quality standards. We need to move our country to the point where the consequences for non-reporting an event or for harming a person are worse than the incentives for staying silent."

In a blunt commentary earlier this year, senior government physicians concluded that "since the pandemic began, U.S. health care safety has declined severely. The fact that the pandemic degraded patient safety so quickly and severely suggests that our health care system lacks a sufficiently resilient safety culture and infrastructure" (Fleisher et al., 2022). To address this very sobering state of affairs impacting our healthcare systems, the Center for Medicare and Medicaid Services (CMS) has discussed renewing their focus, expanding the focus of Patient Safety Indicators, and developing new approaches.

The White House and Congress are discussing the implementation of several initiatives—one of these, a National Patient Safety Board, an independent federal agency modeled on the National Transportation Safety Board, is said by supporters to have lined up Republican and Democratic sponsors in both the House and Senate. Even if legislation is not enacted, bipartisan support increases the odds of public hearings that shine a spotlight on preventable patient safety events (https://npsb.org/).

Hospitals and healthcare organizations must take accountability for the implementation of a safety culture, training of all staff, and communication to support the priority of patient safety (Cohen et al., 2021). Patients deserve to be safe in the hospital and healthcare settings; a culture of patient safety is imperative in health care organizations.

Change starts with awareness. After reading this book, you are now aware of what you must do and actions you can take to keep yourself and your loved ones safe in the healthcare system. I encourage you to get involved in the patient safety movement at any level that speaks to you; we need every voice to bring this national epidemic out of the shadows and shine a megawatt spotlight on this situation.

All my love,
Dr. Julie Siemers

REFERENCES

Introduction

Bonney, W. (2014). Medical errors: moral and ethical considerations. *J Hosp Adm, 3*(2), 80–88.

Millenson, M. L. (2002). Pushing the profession: how the news media turned patient safety into a priority. *Quality in Health Care, 11*(1), 57–63.

Makary, M. A., Daniel, M. (2016) Medical error—the third leading cause of death in the US. *BMJ.* 353:i2139. https://doi.org/10.1136/bmj.i2139

James, J. T. (2013). A New, Evidence-based Estimate of Patient Harms Associated with Hospital Care. *J Patient Safety, 9*(3), 122–128.

Bates, D. W., Levine, D. M., Salmasian, H., Syrowatka, A., Shahian, D. M., Lipsitz, S., Zebrowski, J. P., Myers, L. C., Logan, M. S., Roy, C. G., Iannaccone, C., Frits, M. L., Volk, L. A., Dulgarian, S., Amato, M. G., Edrees, H. H., Sato, L., Folcarelli, P., Einbinder, J. S., . . . Mort, E. (2023). The safety of inpatient health care. *The New England Journal*

of Medicine, 388(2), 142–153. https://doi.org/10.1056/
NEJMsa2206117

de Vries, E. N., Ramrattan, M. A., Smorenburg, S. M., Gouma,
D. J., & Boermeester, M. A. (2008). The incidence and
nature of in-hospital adverse events: a systematic review.
Quality & Safety in Health Care, 17(3), 216. https://doi.org/
10.1136/qshc.2007.023622

Panagiati, M., Khan, K., Keers, R. N., Abuzour, A., Phipps,
D., Kontopantelis, E., Bower, P., Campbell, S., Haneef, R.,
Avery, A. J., & Ashcroft, D. M. (2019). Prevalence, severity,
and nature of preventable patient harm across medical care
settings: systematic review and meta-analysis. *BMJ: British
Medical Journal (Online), 366.* https://doi.org/10.1136/bmj
.l4185

Waldie, J., Tee, S., & Day, T. (2016). Reducing avoidable deaths
from failure to rescue: a discussion paper. *British Journal of
Nursing, 25*(16), 895–900.

Ghazal, L., Saleem, Z., & Amlani, G. (2014). A medical error:
To disclose or not to disclose. *Journal of Clinical Research &
Bioethics, 5*(2), 1.

Fleisher, L. A., Schreiber, M., Cardo, D., & Srinivasan, A. (2022).
Health Care Safety during the Pandemic and Beyond—
Building a System That Ensures Resilience. *The New
England Journal of Medicine, 386*(7), 609–611. https://doi.
org/10.1056/NEJMp2118285

Sutton, E., Brewster, L., & Tarrant, C. (2019). Making infection
prevention and control everyone's business? Hospital staff
views on patient involvement. *Health Expectations, 22*(4),
650–656. https://doi.org/10.1111/hex.12874

Chapter 1

No references

Chapter 2

Martinez, W., Lehmann, L. S., Yue-Yung Hu, Desai, S. P., &
Shapiro, J. (2017). Processes for Identifying and Reviewing

Adverse Events and Near Misses at an Academic Medical Center. *Joint Commission Journal on Quality & Patient Safety, 43*(1), 5–15. https://doi.org/10.1016/j.jcjq.2016.11.001

Van Den Bos, J., Rustagi, K., Gray, T., Halford, M., Ziemkiewicz, E., & Shreve, J. (2015). The $17.1 billion problem: the annual cost of measurable medical errors. *Health Affairs (Project Hope), 30*(4), 596–603. https://doi.org/10.1377/hlthaff.2011.0084

Bonney, W. (2014). Medical errors: moral and ethical considerations. *J Hosp Adm, 32*(32), 80–88.

Sorrell, J. (2017). Ethics: ethical issues with medical errors: shaping a culture of safety in healthcare. *Ojin: The Online Journal of Issues in Nursing, 22*(2). https://doi.org/10.3912/OJIN.Vol22No02EthCol01

Pear, R. (2012). Report finds most errors in hospitals go unreported. https://www.nytimes.com/2012/01/06/health/study-of-medicare-patients-finds-most-hospital-errors-unreported.html

Ahsani-Estahbanati, E., Sergeevich Gordeev, V., & Doshmangir, L. (2022). Interventions to reduce the incidence of medical error and its financial burden in health care systems: A systematic review of systematic reviews. *Frontiers in medicine, 9,* 875426. https://doi.org/10.3389/fmed.2022.875426

Schlachter, L. (2017). *Malpractice: a neurosurgeon reveals how our healthcare system puts patients at risk.* Skyhorse Publishing; 1st edition.

Rodziewicz, T. L., Houseman, B., & Hipskind, J. E. (2022). *Medical Error Reduction and Prevention.* StatPearls Publishing. https://pubmed.ncbi.nlm.nih.gov/29763131/

Bates, D. W., Levine, D. M., Salmasian, H., Syrowatka, A., Shahian, D. M., Lipsitz, S., Zebrowski, J. P., Myers, L. C., Logan, M. S., Roy, C. G., Iannaccone, C., Frits, M. L., Volk, L. A., Dulgarian, S., Amato, M. G., Edrees, H. H., Sato, L., Folcarelli, P., Einbinder, J. S., . . . Mort, E. (2023). The safety of inpatient health care. *The New England Journal of Medicine, 388*(2), 142–153. https://doi.org/10.1056/NEJMsa2206117

Mushta, J., Rush, K. L., & Andersen, E. (2018). Failure to rescue as a nurse-sensitive indicator. *Nursing Forum, 53*(1), 84–92. https://onlinelibrary.wiley.com/doi/10.1111/nuf.12215

Labrague, L. J., Santos, J. A. A., & Fronda, D. C. (2022). Factors associated with missed nursing care and nurse-assessed quality of care during the COVID-19 pandemic. *Journal of Nursing Management, 30*(1), 62. https://doi.org/10.1111/jonm.13483

Patra, K. P., & De Jesus O. (2022), Sentinel Event. StatPearls Publishing. https://www.ncbi.nlm.nih.gov/books/NBK564388/

Dimova, R., Stoyanova, R., & Doykov, I. (2018). Mixed-methods study of reported clinical cases of undesirable events, medical errors, and near misses in health care. *Journal of Evaluation in Clinical Practice, 24*(4), 752–757. https://doi.org/10.1111/jep.12970

Seyma, Z. K., Meral, Y. C., & Atiye, E. (2021). Nurses' Knowledge Levels About the Care of the Patients with Chest Tube. *International Journal of Caring Sciences, 14*(2), 1334–1342.

Chapter 3

Kohn, L. T., Corrigan, J. M., Donaldson, M. S. (2000). *To err is human: building a safer health system*, Institute of Medicine, Washington, DC: National Academy Press. Available from: https://www.ncbi.nlm.nih.gov/books/NBK225182/

Institute of Medicine (2001). *Crossing the quality chasm: A new health system for the 21st century.* Washington, DC: National Academy Press.

Institute of Medicine (2004). *Keeping patients safe: Transforming the work environment of Nurses.* Retrieved from: Keeping Patients Safe: Transforming the Work Environment of Nurses | The National Academies Press (nap.edu)

Millenson, M. L. (2002). Pushing the profession: how the news media turned patient safety into a priority. *Quality in Health Care, 11*(1), 57–63.

Sipherd, R. (2018). Medical errors third-leading cause of death in America. (cnbc.com). https://www.cnbc.com/2018/02/22/medical-errors-third-leading-cause-of-death-in-america.html

Andel, C., Davidow, S. L., Hollander, M. & Moreno, D. A. (2012). The economics of health care quality and medical errors. *J Health Care Finance, 39*(1):39–50.

Rodziewicz, T. L., Houseman, B., & Hipskind, J. E. (2022). *Medical Error Reduction and Prevention.* StatPearls Publishing. https://pubmed.ncbi.nlm.nih.gov/29763131/

Harris, K., Søfteland, E., Moi, A. L., Harthug, S., Storesund, A., Jesuthasan, S., . . . Haugen, A. S. (2020). Patients' and healthcare workers' recommendations for a surgical patient safety checklist—a qualitative study. *England: BioMed Central.* https://doi.org/10.1186/s12913-020-4888-1

Van Den Bos, J., Rustagi, K., Gray, T., Halford, M., Ziemkiewicz, E., & Shreve, J. (2015). The $17.1 billion problem: the annual cost of measurable medical errors. *Health Affairs (Project Hope), 30*(4), 596–603. https://doi.org/10.1377/hlthaff.2011.0084

Bates, D. W., Levine, D. M., Salmasian, H., Syrowatka, A., Shahian, D. M., Lipsitz, S., Zebrowski, J. P., Myers, L. C., Logan, M. S., Roy, C. G., Iannaccone, C., Frits, M. L., Volk, L. A., Dulgarian, S., Amato, M. G., Edrees, H. H., Sato, L., Folcarelli, P., Einbinder, J. S., . . . Mort, E. (2023). The safety of inpatient health care. *The New England Journal of Medicine, 388*(2), 142–153. https://doi.org/10.1056/NEJMsa2206117

Levinson, D. & Department of Health and Human Services (2010). Adverse event in Hospitals: National Incidence among Medicare Beneficiaries. OEI-06-09-00090 (Washington, CD: Office of the Inspector General.) https://oig.hhs.gov/oei/reports/oei-06-09-00090.pdf

Dimova, R., Stoyanova, R., & Doykov, I. (2018). Mixed-methods study of reported clinical cases of undesirable events, medical errors, and near misses in health care. *Journal of Evaluation in Clinical Practice, 24*(4), 752–757. https://doi.org/10.1111/jep.12970

Cohen, S. (2014). Malpractice lawsuits aren't just about the money. https://www.forbes.com/sites/stevecohen/2014/06/18/malpractice-lawsuits-arent-just-about-money/?sh=ba8d311797cd#d2a79162e1b

O'Connor, E., Coates, H. M., Yardley, I. E., & WU, A. W. (2010). Disclosure of patient safety incidents: a comprehensive review. *International Journal for Quality in Health Care, 22*(5), 371–379.

Bonney, W. (2014). Medical errors: moral and ethical considerations. *J Hosp Adm, 32*(32), 80–88.

Ghazal, L., Saleem, Z., & Amlani, G. (2014). A medical error: To disclose or not to disclose. *Journal of Clinical Research & Bioethics, 5*(2), 1.

Africa, L., & Shinners, J. S. (2020). Tracking medical errors and near misses in the new graduate registered nurse. *Nursing Forum, 55*(2), 174–176. https://doi.org/10.1111/nuf.12412

Schlachter, L. (2017). *Malpractice: a neurosurgeon reveals how our healthcare system puts patients at risk*. Skyhorse Publishing; 1st edition.

Kim, Y., & Lee, E. (2020). The relationship between the perception of open disclosure of patient safety incidents, perception of patient safety culture, and ethical awareness in nurses. *BMC Medical Ethics, 21*(1), 104. https://doi.org/10.1186/s12910-020-00546-7

Martinez, W., Lehmann, L. S., Yue-Yung Hu, Desai, S. P., & Shapiro, J. (2017). Processes for Identifying and Reviewing Adverse Events and Near Misses at an Academic Medical Center. *Joint Commission Journal on Quality & Patient Safety, 43*(1), 5–15. https://doi.org/10.1016/j.jcjq.2016.11.001

Chapter 4

Ghazal, L., Saleem, Z., & Amlani, G. (2014). A medical error: To disclose or not to disclose. *Journal of Clinical Research & Bioethics, 5*(2), 1.

Bonney, W. (2014). Medical errors: moral and ethical considerations. *J Hosp Adm, 32*(32), 80–88.

Nong, P., Raj, M., Creary, M., Kardia, S. L. R., & Platt, J. E. (2020). Patient-reported experiences of discrimination in the us health care system. *Jama Network Open, 3*(12), 2029650. https://doi.org/10.1001/jamanetworkopen.2020.29650

Chapter 5

Awdish, R. (2018). *In Shock: My Journey from death to recovery and the redemptive power of hope.* London. Picador— Holtzbrinck Publishing Group.

Schlachter, L. (2017). *Malpractice: a neurosurgeon reveals how our healthcare system puts patients at risk.* Skyhorse Publishing; 1st edition.

Ghazal, L., Saleem, Z., & Amlani, G. (2014). A medical error: To disclose or not to disclose. *Journal of Clinical Research & Bioethics, 5*(2), 1.

Potosky, A. L., Davis, W. W., Hoffman, R. M., Stanford, J. L., Stephenson, R. A., Penson, D. F., & Harlan, L. C. (2004). Five-Year Outcomes After Prostatectomy or Radiotherapy for Prostate Cancer: The Prostate Cancer Outcomes Study. *Journal of the National Cancer Institute, 96*(18), 1358–1367.

Weaver, M. D., Landrigan, C. P., Sullivan, J. P., O'Brien, C. S., Qadri, S., Viyaran, N., Czeisler, C. A., & Barger, L. K. (2023). National improvements in resident physician-reported patient safety after limiting first-year resident physicians' extended duration work shifts: a pooled analysis of prospective cohort studies. *BMJ quality & safety, 32*(2), 81–89. https://doi.org/10.1136/bmjqs-2021-014375

McGlynn, E. A., Asch, S. M., Adams, J., Keesey, J., et al (2003). The quality of health care delivered to adults in the United States. *The New England Journal of Medicine. Boston: 348*(26), 2635–2646.

Recio-Saucedo, A, Dall'Ora, C, Maruotti, A, et al. (2018). What impact does nursing care left undone have on patient outcomes? Review of the literature. *J Clin Nurs. 27*, 2248–2259. https://doi.org/10.1111/jocn.14058

Chapter 6

Burke, J. R., Downey, C., & Almoudaris, A. M. (2022). Failure to Rescue Deteriorating Patients: A Systematic Review of Root Causes and Improvement Strategies, *Journal of Patient Safety, 18*(1). p e140-e155 https://journals.lww.com/journalpatientsafety/abstract/2022/01000/failure_to_rescue_deteriorating_patients__a.28.aspx

Nance, J. (2008). *Why Hospitals Should Fly.* Second River Healthcare; 1st edition.

Acquaviva, K., Haskell, H., & Johnson, J. (2013). Human cognition and the dynamics of Failure to Rescue: The Lewis Blackman Case. *Journal of Professional Nursing, 29*(2), 95–101. https://doi.org/10.1016/j.profnurs.2012.12.009

Chua, W. L., Legido-Quigley, H., Jones, D., Hassan, N. B., Tee, A., & Liaw, S. Y. (2020). A call for better doctor–nurse collaboration: A qualitative study of the experiences of junior doctors and nurses in escalating care for deteriorating ward patients. *Australian Critical Care*, 33(1), p54–61, 8p. Publisher: Elsevier B.V., Database: Supplemental Index

Institute for Healthcare Improvement (2005). Retrieved from http://ihi.org.

Schein, R., Hazday, N., Pena, M., Ruben, B., & Sprung, C. (1990). Clinical antecedents to in-hospital cardiopulmonary arrest. *Chest, 6*(1) 388–92.

Pattni, N., Arzola, C., Malavade, A., Varman,. S., Krimus, L., & Friedman, Z. (2019). Challenging authority and speaking up in the operating room environment: a narrative synthesis. *British Journal of Anaesthesia, 122*(2): 233e244. https://doi. org/10.1016/j.bja.2018.10.056

Bell, S. K., Roche, S. D., Mueller, A., Dente, E., O'Reilly, K., Sarnoff Lee, B., Sands, K., Talmor, D., & Brown, S. M. (2018). Speaking up about care concerns in the ICU: patient and family experiences, attitudes and perceived barriers. *Bmj Quality & Safety, 27*(11), 928–936. https://doi. org/10.1136/bmjqs-2017-007525

Bishop, A. & McDonald, M. (2017). Patient involvement in patient safety: A qualitative study of nursing staff and patient perceptions. *J Patient Safety* 13(2), 82–87

Harris, K., Søfteland, E., Moi, A. L., Harthug, S., Storesund, A., Jesuthasan, S., Sevdalis, N., & Haugen, A. S. (2020). Patients' and healthcare workers' recommendations for a surgical patient safety checklist—a qualitative study. *BMC health services research, 20*(1), 43. https://doi.org/10.1186/ s12913-020-4888-1

Sutton, E., Martin, G., Eborall, H., Tarrant, C. (2023). Undertaking risk and relational work to manage vulnerability: Acute medical patients' involvement in patient safety in the NHS, *Social Science & Medicine, Volume 320,* 115729, ISSN 0277-9536, https://doi.org/10.1016/j.socscimed.2023.115729.

Chapter 7

Zimmermann, P. G. (2008). Preventing lawsuits by noting and acting on key aspects in a patient's condition. *Orthopaedic Nursing, 27*(1), 31–7.

Lavoie, P., Pepin, J., & Alderson, M. (2014). Defining patient deterioration through acute care and intensive care nurses' perspectives. *Nursing in Critical Care, 21*(2), 68–77. https:// doi.org/10.1111/nicc.12114

Jones, S., Bottle, A., & Griffiths, P. (2011). *An assessment of "failure to rescue" derived from routing NHS data as a nursing sensitive patient safety indicator for surgical* *inpatient care.*National Nursing Research Unit. King's College London.

Levett-Jones, T., Hoffman, K., Dempsey, J., Jeong, Y. S., Noble, D., Norton, C. A., et al. (2010). The 'five rights' of clinical reasoning: An educational model to enhance nursing students' ability to identify and manage clinically 'at risk' patients. *Nurse Education Today,* 30, 515–520.

Garvey, P. (2015). Failure to rescue: The nurse's impact. *Medsurg Nursing, 24*(3), 145–149.

Hodgetts, T. J., Kenward, G., Vlackonikolis, I., Payne, S., & Castle, N., Crouch, R., & . . . Shaikh, L. (2002). Incidence, location and reasons for avoidable in-hospital cardiac arrest in district general hospital. *Resuscitation, 54*(2), 115–123. https://doi.org/10.1016/S0300-9572(02)00098-9

Simmonds T. C. (2005). Best-practice protocols: implementing a rapid response system of care. *Nursing management, 36*(7), 41–59. https://doi.org/10.1097/00006247-200507000-00010

Thielen, J. (2014). Failure to rescue as the conceptual basis for nursing clinical peer review. *Journal of Nursing Care Quality, 29*(2), 155–163. https://journals.lww.com/jncqjournal/abstract/2014/04000/failure_to_rescue_as_the_conceptual_basis_for.9.aspx

Fasolino, T., & Verdin, T. (2015). Nursing Surveillance and Physiological Signs of Deterioration. *MEDSURG Nursing, 24*(6), 397–402.

Mushta, J., Rush, K. L., & Andersen, E. (2018). Failure to rescue as a nurse-sensitive indicator. *Nursing Forum, 53*(1), 84–92. https://doi.org/10.1111/nuf.12215

Panday, R. S. N., Minderhoud, T. C., Alam, N., Nanayakarra, P. W. B. (2017). Prognostic value of early warning scores in the emergency department (ED) and acute medical unit (AMU): A narrative review. *Eur. J. Intern. Med. 45*, 20–31. https://www.ejinme.com/article/S0953-6205(17)30375-8/fulltext

Farhat, A. (2008). Rapid response teams prove value for safety of your patients. *Healthcare Risk Management, 30*(1), 1–12.

Roney, J., Whitley, B., Maples, J., Futrell, L., Stunkard, K., & Long, J. (2015). Modified early warning scoring (MEWS): Evaluating the evidence for tool inclusion of sepsis screening criteria and impact on mortality and failure to rescue. *Journal of Clinical Nursing, 24*(23-24), 3343–3354. https://doi.org/10.1111/jocn.12952

Herron, E. K. (2017). New graduate nurses' preparation for recognition and prevention of failure to rescue: A qualitative study. *Journal of Clinical Nursing, 27*(1-2), 401. https://doi.org/10.1111/jocn.14016

Labrague, L. J., Santos, J. A. A., & Fronda, D. C. (2022). Factors associated with missed nursing care and nurse-assessed quality of care during the COVID-19 pandemic. *Journal of Nursing Management, 30*(1), 62. https://doi.org/10.1111/jonm.13483

Considine, J., & Currey, J. (2015). Ensuring a proactive, evidence-based, patient safety approach to patient assessment. *Journal of clinical nursing, 24*(1-2), 300–307. https://doi.org/10.1111/jocn.12641

Ghaferi, A. (2017). Despite Clues, Failed to Rescue. AHRQ Patient Safety Network. Retrieved from: https://psnet.ahrq.gov/web-mm/despite-clues-failed-rescue

Burke, J. R., Downey, C., & Almoudaris, A. M. (2022). Failure to Rescue Deteriorating Patients: A Systematic Review of Root Causes and Improvement Strategies, *Journal of Patient Safety, 18*(1). p c140 e155. https://journals.lww.com/journalpatientsafety/abstract/2022/01000/failure_to_rescue_deteriorating_patients__a.28.aspx

Meyer, G. A., Lavin, M. A., & Perry, A. G. (2007). Is it time for a new category of nursing diagnosis?. International journal of nursing terminologies and classifications : the official journal of NANDA International, 18(2), 45–50. https://doi.org/10.1111/j.1744-618X.2007.00049.x

Dalton, M., Harrison, J., Malin, A., & Leavey, C. (2018). Factors that influence nurses' assessment of patient acuity and response to acute deterioration. *British Journal of Nursing,* *27*(4), 212–218. https://doi.org/10.12968/bjon.2018.27.4.212

Brekke, I. J., Puntervoll, L. H., Pedersen, P. B., Kellett, J., & Brabrand, M. (2019). The value of vital sign trends in predicting and monitoring clinical deterioration: A systematic review. *PloS One, 14*(1), e0210875. http://doi.org/10.1371/journal.pone.0210875

Ashcraft, A. (2004). Differentiating between pre-arrest and failure to rescue. *MEDSURG Nursing 13,*(4).

Institute for Healthcare Improvement (2005). Retrieved from http://ihi.org.

Andrews, T., & Waterman, H. (2005). Packaging: a grounded theory of how to report physiological deterioration effectively. *Journal of Advanced Nursing, 52*(5), 473–81.

Rutherford P, Lee B, Greiner A. (2004). Transforming Care at the Bedside. *IHI Innovation Series white paper. Boston: Institute for Healthcare Improvement.* (Available on www.IHI.org)

Wood, C., Chaboyer, W., & Carr, P. (2019). How do nurses use early warning scoring systems to detect and act on patient deterioration to ensure patient safety? A scoping review. *International Journal of Nursing Studies, 94,* 166–178. https://doi.org/10.1016/j.ijnurstu.2019.03.012

Reed, K. & May, R. (2011). HealthGrades Patient Safety in American Hospitals Study. Retrieved from https://patientsafetymovement.org/

ECRI (2019). ECRI names top 10 patient safety concerns for 2019. Retrieved from: https://hitconsultant.net/2019/03/15/top-10-patient-safety-concerns-2019/

Hughes, M. (2004). Processes contributing to failure to rescue in acute care hospitals. *Abstract Academy Health Meeting, 21*(1831). Retrieve pdf from https://www.lifescitrc.org/download.cfm?submissionID=6011

Cioffi, J. (2000). Nurses' experience of making decision to call emergency assistance to their patients. *Journal of Advanced Nursing, 32*(1), 108–114.

Cooper, S., Beauchamp, A., Bogossian, F., Bucknall, T., Cant, R., DeVries, B., . . . Young, S. (2012). Managing patient deterioration: a protocol for enhancing undergraduate nursing students' competence through web-based simulation and feedback techniques. *BMC Nursing, 11*(1), 18–24. https://doi-org.chamberlainuniversity.idm.oclc.org/10.1186/1472-6955-11-18

Cooper, S., Cant, R., Porter, J., Missen, K., Sparkes, L., McConnell-Henry, T., & Endacott, R. (2013). Managing patient deterioration: assessing teamwork and individual performance. *Emergency Medicine Journal, 30*(5), 377–381. https://doi.org/10.1136/emermed-2012-201312

Schein, R., Hazday, N., Pena, M., Ruben, B., & Sprung, C. (1990). Clinical antecedents to in-hospital cardiopulmonary arrest. *Chest, 6*(1) 388–92.

Hart, P. L., Spiva, L. A., Baio, P., Huff, B., Whitfield, D., Law, T., Wells, T., & Mendoza, I. G. (2014). Medical-surgical nurses' perceived self-confidence and leadership abilities as first responders in acute patient deterioration events. *Journal of Clinical Nursing, 23*(19-20), 2769–2778. https://doi.org/10.1111/jocn.12523

Kyriacos, U., Jelsma, J., & Jordan, S. (2011). Monitoring vital signs using early warning scoring systems: A review of the literature. *Journal of Nursing Management, 19*(3), 311 330. https://doi.org/10.1111/j.1365-2834.2011.01246.x

Allen, G. (2020). Barriers to non-critical care nurses identifying and responding to early signs of clinical deterioration in acute care facilities. *MEDSURG Nursing, 29*(1), 43–52.

Herron, E. K. (2017). New graduate nurses' preparation for recognition and prevention of failure to rescue: A qualitative study. *Journal of Clinical Nursing, 27*(1-2), 401. https://doi.org/10.1111/jocn.14016

Hart, P. L., Spiva, L., Dolly, L., Lang-Coleman, K., & Prince-Williams, N. (2016). Medical-surgical nurses' experiences as first responders during deterioration events: A qualitative study. *Journal of Clinical Nursing, 25*(21-22), 3241–3251. https://doi.org/10.1111/jocn.13357

Waldie, J., Tee, S., & Day, T. (2016a). Reducing avoidable deaths from failure to rescue: a discussion paper. *British Journal of Nursing, 25*(16), 895–900.

Van Den Bos, J., Rustagi, K., Gray, T., Halford, M., Ziemkiewicz, E., & Shreve, J. (2015). The $17.1 billion problem: the annual cost of measurable medical errors. *Health Affairs (Project Hope), 30*(4), 596–603. https://doi.org/10.1377/hlthaff.2011.0084

Silber, J. H., Williams, S. V., Krakauer, H., Schwartz, J. S. (1992). Hospital and patient characteristics associated with death after surgery. A study of adverse occurrence and failure to rescue. *Med Care, 30*(7):615–629. https://journals.lww.com/lww-medicalcare/abstract/1992/07000/hospital_and_patient_characteristics_associated.4.aspx

Verillo, S. C., & Winters, B. D. (2018). Review: Continuous Monitoring to Detect Failure to Rescue in Adult Postoperative Inpatients. *Biomedical Instrumentation & Technology, 52*(4), 281–287.

Ryan H., Cadman C, & Hann L. (2004). Critical care. Setting standards for assessment of ward patients at risk of deterioration. *British Journal of Nursing, 13*(20), 1186–1190. https://doi.org/10.12968/bjon.2004.13.20.17008

Preston, R. M., & Flynn, D. J. (2010). Observations in acute care: Evidence-based approach to patient safety. *British Journal of Nursing, 19*(7), 442–447.

Subbe, C. P., & Welch, J. R. (2013). Failure to rescue: using rapid response systems to improve care of the deteriorating patient in hospital. *Clinical Risk, 19*(1), 6–11. https://doi.org/10.1177/1356262213486451

Chapter 8

Quirke, S., Coombs, M., McEldowney, R. (2011). Suboptimal care of the acutely unwell ward patient: a concept analysis. *Journal of Advanced Nursing, 67*(8), p. 1834–1845. https://doi.org/10.1111/j.1365-2648.2011.05664.x

Hart, P. L., Spiva, L., Dolly, L., Lang-Coleman, K., & Prince-Williams, N. (2016). Medical-surgical nurses' experiences as first responders during deterioration events: A qualitative study. *Journal of Clinical Nursing, 25*(21-22), 3241–3251. https://doi.org/10.1111/jocn.13357

Chua, W. L., Mackey, S., Ng, E. K. C., & Liaw, S. Y. (2013). Front line nurses' experiences with deteriorating ward patients: a qualitative study. *International Nursing Review, 60*(4), 501–509. https://doi.org/10.1111/inr.12061

Chua, W. L., Legido-Quigley, H., Jones, D., Hassan, N. B., Tee, A., & Liaw, S. Y. (2020). A call for better doctor–nurse collaboration: A qualitative study of the experiences of junior doctors and nurses in escalating care for deteriorating ward patients. *Australian Critical Care*, 33(1), p54–61, 8p. Publisher: Elsevier B.V., Database: Supplemental Index

Panday, R. S. N., Minderhoud, T. C., Alam, N., Nanayakarra, P. W. B. (2017). Prognostic value of early warning scores in the emergency department (ED) and acute medical unit (AMU): A narrative review. *Eur. J. Intern. Med. 45*, 20–31. https://doi.org/10.1016/j.ejim.2017.09.027.

Verillo, S. C., & Winters, B. D. (2018). Review: Continuous Monitoring to Detect Failure to Rescue in Adult Postoperative Inpatients. *Biomedical Instrumentation & Technology, 52*(4), 281–287. https://doi-org.chamberlain university.idm.oclc.org/10.2345/0899-8205-52.4.281

Kavanagh, J. & Szweda, C. (2017). A crisis in competency: The strategic and ethical imperative to assessing new graduate Nurses' clinical reasoning. *Nursing Education Perspectives, 38*(2). https://journals.lww.com/neponline/

abstract/2017/03000/a_crisis_in_competency__the_
strategic_and_ethical.3.aspx

Jackson, S. (2017). Rapid response teams: What's the latest?. *Nursing, 47*, 34–41. https://doi.org/10.1097/01.NURSE. 0000526885.10306.21

Shearer, B., Marshall, S., Buist, M. D., Finnigan, M., Kitto, S., Hore, T., . . . Ramsay, W. (2012). What stops hospital clinical staff from following protocols? an analysis of the incidence and factors behind the failure of bedside clinical staff to activate the rapid response system in a multi-campus Australian metropolitan healthcare service. *BMJ Quality & Safety, 21*(7), 569. doi:http:// dx.doi.org.chamberlainuniversity.idm.oclc.org/10.1136/ bmjqs-2011-000692

Sharek, P. J. (2008). Rapid response teams prove value for safety of your patients. *Healthcare Risk Management, 30*(1), 1–12.

Rischer, K. (2022). *Think Like a Nurse: Developing Clinical Judgment for Successful Professional Practice.*

Olsen, S. L., Nedrebø, B., Strand, K. et al. (2023). Reduction in omission events after implementing a Rapid Response System: a mortality review in a department of gastrointestinal surgery. *BMC Health Serv Res 23*, 179. https://doi. org/10.1186/s12913-023-09159-3

Olsen, S. L., Søreide, E., Hansen, B. S. (2022). We Are Not There Yet: A Qualitative System Probing Study of a Hospital Rapid Response System, *Journal of Patient Safety,* 10, 10.1097/PTS.0000000000001000. https://journals.lww. com/journalpatientsafety/abstract/2021/12000/tackling_ ambulatory_safety_risks_through_patient.22.aspx

Needham, D., Thompson, D., Holzmueller, C., Dorman, T., Lubomski, L., Wu, A., . . . Pronovost, P. (2004). A system factors analysis of airway events from the intensive care unit safety reporting system (ICUSRS). *Critical Care Medicine, 32*(11), 2227–2233. https://journals.lww.com/

ccmjournal/abstract/2004/11000/a_system_factors_
analysis_of_airway_events_from.7.aspx

Crewdson, K., Lockey, D. J., Raislien, J., Lossius, H. M., & Rehn, M. (2017). The success of pre-hospital tracheal intubation by different pre-hospital providers: a systematic literature review and meta-analysis. *Critical Care, 21*(1). https://doi.org/10.1186/s13054-017-1603-7

Cook, T. M., & MacDougall-Davis, S. R. (2012). *Complications and failure of airway management* doi:https://doi-org.chamberlainuniversity.idm.oclc.org/10.1093/bja/aes393

da Silva, Paulo Sergio Lucas, & Fonseca, M. C. M. (2012). Unplanned endotracheal extubations in the intensive care unit: Systematic review, critical appraisal, and evidence-based recommendations. *Anesthesia and analgesia, 114*(5), 1003–1014. https://doi.org/10.1213/ANE.0b013e31824b0296

Chapter 9

Numminen, O., Leino-Kilpi, H., Isoaho, H., & Meretoja, R. (2015). Ethical climate and nurse competence—newly graduated nurses' perceptions. *Nursing Ethics, 22*(8), 845–859. https://doi.org/10.1177/0969733014557137

Clarke-Pearson, D. L., & Geller, E. J. (2013). Complications of hysterectomy. *Obstetrics and Gynecology, 121*(3), 654–673. https://doi.org/10.1097/AOG.0b013e3182841594

Benner, P. E. (2010). *Educating nurses: a call for radical transformation* (1st ed., Ser. The jossey bass higher and adult education series). Jossey-Bass.

Meyer, G., & Ann Lavin, M. (2005). Vigilance: The Essence of Nursing. *Journal of Nurse Life Care Planning, 13*(3), 100–111. https://doi.org/10.3912/OJIN.Vol10No03PPT01

Saintsing, D., Gibson, L. M., & Pennington, A. W. (2011). The novice nurse and clinical decision-making: How to avoid errors. *Journal of Nursing Management, 19*(3), 354–359. https://doi.org/10.1111/j.1365-2834.2011.01248.x

Wangensteen, S., Johansson, I. S., Björkström, M. E., & Nordström, G. (2012). Newly graduated nurses' perception of competence and possible predictors: a cross-sectional survey. *Journal of professional nursing : official journal of the American Association of Colleges of Nursing, 28*(3), 170–181. https://doi.org/10.1016/j.profnurs.2011.11.014

Nursing Solutions Incorporated (20210. National health care retention & RN staffing report. 2021 Mar [cited 2021 Dec https://www.nsinursingsolutions.com/Documents/Library/NSI_National_Health_Care_Retention_Report.pdf

Wong, B. M., Baum, K. D., Headrick, L. A., Holmboe, E. S., Moss, F., Ogrinc, G., Shojania, K. G., Vaux, E., Warm, E. J., & Frank, J. R. (2020). Building the Bridge to Quality: An Urgent Call to Integrate Quality Improvement and Patient Safety Education with Clinical Care. Academic medicine : *Journal of the Association of American Medical Colleges, 95*(1), 59–68. https://doi.org/10.1097/ACM.0000000000002937

Kavanagh, J. & Szweda, C. (2017). A crisis in competency: The strategic and ethical imperative to assessing new graduate Nurses' clinical reasoning. *Nursing Education Perspectives, 38*(2). https://journals.lww.com/neponline/abstract/2017/03000/a_crisis_in_competency__the_strategic_and_ethical.3.aspx

Kavanagh, J. M. & Sharpnack, P. A. (2021). "Crisis in Competency: A Defining Moment in Nursing Education". *The Online Journal of Issues in Nursing, 26*(1), Manuscript 2. https://doi.org/10.3912/OJIN.Vol26No01Man02

Huston, C. (2013). The Impact of Emerging Technology on Nursing Care: Warp Speed Ahead. Online *Journal of Issues in Nursing, 18*(2), 1. https://doi.org/10.3912/OJIN.Vol18No02Man01

Waldie, J., Tee, S., & Day, T. (2016). Reducing avoidable deaths from failure to rescue: a discussion paper. *British Journal of Nursing, 25*(16), 895–900.

Herron, E. K. (2017). New graduate nurses' preparation for recognition and prevention of failure to rescue: A qualitative study. *Journal of Clinical Nursing, 27*(1-2), 401. https://doi.org/10.1111/jocn.14016

Verillo, S. C., & Winters, B. D. (2018). Review: Continuous Monitoring to Detect Failure to Rescue in Adult Postoperative Inpatients. *Biomedical Instrumentation & Technology, 52*(4), 281–287. https://doi-org.chamberlain university.idm.oclc.org/10.2345/0899-8205-52.4.281

Bowden, V., Bradas, C., & McNett, M. (2019). Impact of level of nurse experience on falls in medical surgical units. *Journal of Nursing Management, 27*(4), 833–839. https://doi.org/10.1111/jonm.12742

Hart, P. L., Spiva, L., Dolly, L., Lang-Coleman, K., & Prince-Williams, N. (2016). Medical-surgical nurses' experiences as first responders during deterioration events: A qualitative study. *Journal of Clinical Nursing, 25*(21-22), 3241–3251. https://doi.org/10.1111/jocn.13357

Cooper, S., Kinsman, L., Buykx, P., McConnell-Henry, T., Endacott, R., & Scholes, J. (2010). Managing the deteriorating patient in a simulated environment: nursing students' knowledge, skill and situation awareness. *Journal of Clinical Nursing, 19*, 2309–2318.

Africa, L., & Shinners, J. S. (2020). Tracking medical errors and near misses in the new graduate registered nurse. *Nursing Forum, 55*(2), 174–176. https://doi.org/10.1111/nuf.12412

Hodgetts, T. J., Kenward, G., Vlackonikolis, I., Payne, S., & Castle, N., Crouch, R., & . . . Shaikh, L. (2002b). Incidence, location and reasons for avoidable in-hospital cardiac arrest in district general hospital. *Resuscitation, 54*(2), 115–123. https://doi.org/10.1016/S0300-9572(02)00098-9

Hart, P. L., Spiva, L., Dolly, L., Lang-Coleman, K., & Prince-Williams, N. (2016). Medical-surgical nurses' experiences as first responders during deterioration events: A qualitative study. *Journal of Clinical Nursing, 25*(21-22), 3241–3251. https://doi.org/10.1111/jocn.13357

Aiken, L. H., Shange, J., Xue, Y., & Sloane, D. M. (2013). Hospital use of agency-employed supplemental nurses and patient mortality and failure to rescue. *Health Services Research, 48*(3), 931–948. https://doi.org/10.1111/1475-6773 .12018

Kim, Y., & Lee, E. (2020). The relationship between the perception of open disclosure of patient safety incidents, perception of patient safety culture, and ethical awareness in nurses. *BMC Medical Ethics, 21*(1), 104. https://doi. org/10.1186/s12910-020-00546-7

Hall, L. M., Doran, D., & Pink, G. H. (2004). Nurse Staffing Models, Nursing Hours, and Patient Safety Outcomes. *The Journal of Nursing Administration, 34*(1), 41–45. https:// journals.lww.com/jonajournal/abstract/2004/01000/nurse _staffing_models,_nursing_hours,_and_patient.9.aspx

Snavely, T. M. (2016). A brief economic analysis of the looming nursing shortage in the United States. *Nursing Economic, 34*(2), 98. Retrieved from https://www.ncbi.nlm.nih.gov/ pubmed/27265953

Clarke, S., & Aiken, L. (2003). Failure to rescue: Needless deaths are prime examples of the need for more nurses at the bedside. *American Journal of Nursing 103*(1), 42–47. https:// journals.lww.com/ajnonline/citation/2003/01000/failure_to_ rescue__needless_deaths_are_prime.20.aspx

Ashcraft, A. (2004). Differentiating between pre-arrest and failure to rescue. *MEDSURG Nursing 13*(4), 211–216.

Audet, L.-A., Bourgault, P., & Rochefort, C. M. (2018). Associations between nurse education and experience and the risk of mortality and adverse events in acute care hospitals: A systematic review of observational studies. *International Journal of Nursing Studies, 80*, 128–146. https://doi.org/10.1016/j.ijnurstu.2018.01.007

Ryan H., Cadman C, & Hann L. (2004). Critical care. Setting

standards for assessment of ward patients at risk of deterioration. *British Journal of Nursing, 13*(20), 1186–1190. https://doi.org/10.12968/bjon.2004.13.20.17008

Henson, J. S. (2020). Burnout or Compassion Fatigue: A Comparison of Concepts. *MEDSURG Nursing, 29*(2), 77–95.

Nursing Solutions Incorporated (20210. National health care retention & RN staffing report. 2021 Mar [cited 2021 Dec] https://www.nsinursingsolutions.com/Documents/Library/NSI_National_Health_Care_Retention_Report.pdf

MacKusick, C. I., & Minick, P. (2010). Why are nurses leaving? Findings from an initial qualitative study on nursing attrition. *Medsurg nursing : official journal of the Academy of Medical-Surgical Nurses, 19*(6), 335–340.

Chua, W. L., Legido-Quigley, H., Ng, P. Y., McKenna, L., Hassan, N. B., & Liaw, S. Y. (2019). Seeing the whole picture in enrolled and registered nurses' experiences in recognizing clinical deterioration in general ward patients: A qualitative study. *International Journal of Nursing Studies, 95*, 56–64. https://doi.org/10.1016/j.ijnurstu.2019.04.012

Phillips, J. A., & Miltner, R. (2015). Work hazards for an aging nursing workforce. *Journal of Nursing Management, 23*, 803–812. https://doi.org/10.1111/jonm.12217

Goodacre, P. (2017). Literature review: Why do we continue to lose our nurses? *Australian Journal of Advanced Nursing (Online), 34*(4), 50–56.

Jarrad, R. A., & Hammad, S. (2020). Oncology nurses' compassion fatigue, burn out and compassion satisfaction. *Annals of General Psychiatry, 19*(1), 1–8. https://doi.org/10.1186/s12991-020-00272-9

Halbesleben, J. R. B., Wakefield, B. J., Wakefield, D. S., & Cooper, L. B. (2008). Nurse burnout and patient safety outcomes: nurse safety perception versus reporting behavior. *Western Journal of Nursing Research, 30*(5), 560–577. https://doi.org/10.1177/0193945907311322

Dimova, R., Stoyanova, R., & Doykov, I. (2018). Mixed-methods study of reported clinical cases of undesirable events, medical errors, and near misses in health care. *Journal of Evaluation in Clinical Practice, 24*(4), 752–757. https://doi. org/10.1111/jep.12970

James-Scotter, M., Walker, C., & Jacobs, S. (2019). An interprofessional perspective on job satisfaction in the operating room: a review of the literature. *Journal of Interprofessional Care, 33*(6), 782–794. https://doi-org.westcoastuniversity. idm.oclc.org/10.1080/13561820.2019.1593118

Park, J. Y., & Hwang, J. I. (2021). [relationships among non-nursing tasks, nursing care left undone, nurse outcomes and medical errors in integrated nursing care wards in small and medium-sized general hospitals]. *Journal of Korean Academy of Nursing, 51*(1), 27–39. https://doi.org/10.4040/ jkan.20201

Chapter 10

Mok, W., Wang, W., & Liaw, S. (2015). Vital signs monitoring to detect patient deterioration: An integrative literature review. *International Journal of Nursing Practice, 21*, 91–98. https:// doi.org/10.1111/ijn.12329

Brekke, I. J., Puntervoll, L. H., Pedersen, P. B., Kellett, J., & Brabrand, M. (2019). The value of vital sign trends in predicting and monitoring clinical deterioration: A systematic review. *PloS One, 14*(1), e0210875. http:doi.org/10.1371/ journal.pone.0210875

Ryan H., Cadman C, & Hann L. (2004). Critical care. Setting standards for assessment of ward patients at risk of deterioration. *British Journal of Nursing, 13*(20), 1186–1190. https:// doi.org/10.12968/bjon.2004.13.20.17008

Hillman, K., Chen, J., Cretikos, M., Bellomo, R. (2005). Introduction of the medical emergency team (MET) system: a cluster randomized controlled trial. *The Lancet, 365*(9477), 2091–2097.

Hogan, J. (2006). Respiratory assessment. Why don't nurses

monitor the respiratory rates of patients? *British Journal of Nursing (BJN)*, 15(9), 489–492.

Allen, G. (2020). Barriers to non-critical care nurses identifying and responding to early signs of clinical deterioration in acute care facilities. *MEDSURG Nursing*, 29(1), 43–52.

Subbe, C. P., & Welch, J. R. (2013). Failure to rescue: using rapid response systems to improve care of the deteriorating patient in hospital. *Clinical Risk*, 19(1), 6–11. https://doi. org/10.1177/1356262213486451

Chua, W. L., Mackey, S., Ng, E. K. C., & Liaw, S. Y. (2013). Front line nurses' experiences with deteriorating ward patients: a qualitative study. *International Nursing Review*, 60(4), 501–509. https://doi.org/10.1111/inr.12061

Smith, I., Mackay, J., Fahrid, N., & Krucheck, D. (2011). *Respiratory rate measurement: A comparison of methods.* Mark Allen Holdings Limited. https://doi.org/10.12968/ bjha.2011.5.1.18

Garvey, P. (2015). Failure to rescue: The nurse's impact. *Medsurg Nursing*, 24(3), 145–149.

Smith, M. B., Chiovaro, J. C., O'Neil, M., Kansagara, D., Quiñones, A. R., Freeman, M., & . . . Slatore, C. G. (2014). Early warning system scores for clinical deterioration in hospitalized patients: a systematic review. *Annals of the American Thoracic Society*, 11(9), 1454–1465. https://doi. org/10.1513/AnnalsATS.201403-102OC

Panday, R. S. N., Minderhoud, T. C., Alam, N., Nanayakarra, P. W. B. (2017). Prognostic value of early warning scores in the emergency department (ED) and acute medical unit (AMU): A narrative review. *Eur. J. Intern. Med. 45*, 20–31. https://doi.org/10.1016/j.ejim.2017.09.027.

Parkes, R. (2011). Rate of respiration: The forgotten vital sign. *Emergency Nurse : The Journal of the RCN Accident and Emergency Nursing Association*, 19(2), 12. https://journals. rcni.com//doi/abs/10.7748/en2011.05.19.2.12.c8504

Roberts, L., Lanes, S., Kyte, J., Grady, J., Holdship, J., Carey, C.,

Cooney, K., & Ramessur, S. (2022). Acute pain assessments and records: a pilot study of digital transformation. *British Journal of Nursing, 31*(10), 541–548. https://doi.org/10.12968/bjon.2022.31.10.541

Chapter 11

Zimmermann, P. G. (2008). Preventing lawsuits by noting and acting on key aspects in a patient's condition. *Orthopaedic Nursing, 27*(1), 31–7.

Hogan, J. (2006). Respiratory assessment. Why don't nurses monitor the respiratory rates of patients? *British Journal of Nursing (BJN)*, 15(9), 489–492.

Considine, J. and Currey, J. (2015), Ensuring a proactive, evidence-based, patient safety approach to patient assessment. *J Clin Nurs, 24*: 300–307.

Benner, P. (1984). *From novice to expert: Excellence and power in clinical nursing practice.* Menlo Park, CA: Addison-Wesley Publishing Co., Nursing Division.

Rischer, K. (2022). *Think Like a Nurse: Developing Clinical Judgment for Successful Professional Practice.*

Chua, W. L., Legido-Quigley, H., Ng, P. Y., McKenna, L., Hassan, N. B., & Liaw, S. Y. (2019). Seeing the whole picture in enrolled and registered nurses' experiences in recognizing clinical deterioration in general ward patients: A qualitative study. *International Journal of Nursing Studies, 95*, 56–64. https://doi.org/10.1016/j.ijnurstu.2019.04.012

Lima, S., Newall, F., Kinney, S., Jordan, H. L., & Hamilton, B. (2014). How competent are they? graduate nurses self-assessment of competence at the start of their careers. *Collegian, 21*(4), 353–358. https://doi.org/10.1016/j.colegn.2013.09.001

Van Den Bos, J., Rustagi, K., Gray, T., Halford, M., Ziemkiewicz, E., & Shreve, J. (2015). The $17.1 billion problem: the annual cost of measurable medical errors. *Health Affairs (Project*

Hope), 30(4), 596–603. https://doi.org/10.1377/hlthaff.2011
.0084

Padula, W. V., & Delarmente, B. A. (2019). The national cost
of hospital-acquired pressure injuries in the united states.
International Wound Journal, 16(3), 634–640. https://doi.
org/10.1111/iwj.13071

Fleisher, L. A., Schreiber, M., Cardo, D., & Srinivasan, A. (2022).
Health Care Safety during the Pandemic and Beyond—
Building a System That Ensures Resilience. *The New
England Journal of Medicine, 386*(7), 609–611. https://doi.
org/10.1056/NEJMp2118285

Verillo, S. C., & Winters, B. D. (2018). Review: Continuous
Monitoring to Detect Failure to Rescue in Adult
Postoperative Inpatients. *Biomedical Instrumentation &
Technology, 52*(4), 281–287. https://doi-org.chamberlain
university.idm.oclc.org/10.2345/0899-8205-52.4.281

Kaw, R., Pasupuleti, V., Walker, E. (2012). Postoperative complications in patients with obstructive sleep apnea. *Chest
141*(2):436–41.

Kjorven, M., Dunton, D., Milo, R., & Gerein, L. (2011). Bedside
capnography: better management of surgical patients with
obstructive sleep apnea. *The Canadian Nurse, 107*(9), 24–26.

ECRI Institute (2017). Top 10 Hospital C-Suite WATCH LIST.
ECRI Institute. Available at: https://www.ecri.org/Pages/
ECRI-Institute-2017-Top-10-Hospital-C-Suite-Watch-List.
aspx

Blouw, E., Rudolph, A., Narr, B., & Sarr, M. (2003). The frequency of respiratory failure in patients with morbid obesity
undergoing gastric bypass. *AANA Journal, 71*(1), 45–50.

Valderas, J. M., Starfield, B., Sibbald, B., Salisbury, C., Roland,
M. (2009). Defining comorbidity: implications for
understanding health and health services. *Ann Fam Med.*
7(4):357–63. PMID: 19597174; PMCID: PMC2713155. https://
doi.org/10.1370/afm.983

Koyyada, R., Nagalla, B., Tummala, A., Singh, A. D., Patnam, S., Barigala, R., Kandala, M., Krishna, V., & Manda, S. V. (2022). Prevalence and Impact of Preexisting Comorbidities on Overall Clinical Outcomes of Hospitalized COVID-19 Patients. *BioMed Research International*, 1–12. https://doi.org/10.1155/2022/2349890

Hirter, J., & Van Nest, R. L. (1995). Vigilance: A concept and a reality. *CRNA: The Clinical Forum for Nurse Anesthetists*, 6(2), 96–98.

Meyer, G., & Ann Lavin, M. (2005). Vigilance: The Essence of Nursing. *Journal of Nurse Life Care Planning*, 13(3), 100–111. https://doi.org/10.3912/OJIN.Vol10No03PPT01

Chapter 12

Schmier, J. K., Hulme-Lowe, C. K., Semenova, S., Klenk, J. A., DeLeo, P. C., Sedlak, R., & Carlson, P. A. (2016). Estimated hospital costs associated with preventable health care-associated infections if health care antiseptic products were unavailable. *ClinicoEconomics and Outcomes Research*, 1, 197–205.

Sutton, E., Brewster, L., & Tarrant, C. (2019). Making infection prevention and control everyone's business? Hospital staff views on patient involvement. *Health Expectations*, 22(4), 650–656. https://doi.org/10.1111/hex.12874

Ban, K. A., Minei, J. P., Laronga, C., Harbrecht, B. G., Jensen, E. H., Fry, D. E., Itani, K. M., Dellinger, E. P., Ko, C. Y., Duane, T. M. (2017). American College of Surgeons and Surgical Infection Society: Surgical Site Infection Guidelines, 2016 Update. *J Am Coll Surg*. 224(1):59–74. Epub 2016 Nov 30. PMID: 27915053. https://journals.lww.com/journalacs/citation/2017/01000/american_college_of_surgeons_and_surgical.8.aspx

Balu, P., Ravikumar, D., Somasunder, V. M., Suga, S. S. D., Sivagananam, P., Jeyasheelan, V. P., Sreekandan, R. N., James, K. M., Bopaiah, S. K., Chelladurai, U. M., Kumar,

M. R., Chellapandian, P., Sundharesan, N., Krishnan, M., Kunasekaran, V., Kumaravel, K., Manickaraj, R. G. J., Veeraraghvan, V. P., & Mohan, S. K. (2021). Assessment of Knowledge, Attitude and Practice on Prevention of Catheter-associated Urinary Tract Infection (CAUTI) among Health Care Professionals Working in a Tertiary Care Teaching Hospital. *Journal of Pure & Applied Microbiology, 15*(1), 335–345. https://doi.org/10.22207/JPAM.15.1.28

Barnes, S. (2018). Surgical Site Infection prevention in 2018 and beyond. *AORN, 107*(5), p547–550, 4p. Publisher: Wiley-Blackwell., Database: Supplemental Index.

Fleisher, L. A., Schreiber, M., Cardo, D., & Srinivasan, A. (2022). Health Care Safety during the Pandemic and Beyond— Building a System That Ensures Resilience. *The New England Journal of Medicine, 386*(7), 609–611. https://doi.org/10.1056/NEJMp2118285

Buetti, N., Marschall, J., Drees, M., Fakih, M., Hadaway, L., Maragakis, L., . . . Mermel, L. (2022). Strategies to prevent central line-associated bloodstream infections in acute-care hospitals: 2022 Update. *Infection Control & Hospital Epidemiology, 43*(5), 553–569. https://doi.org/10.1017/ice.2022.87

Jones, B. E., Sarvet, A. L., Ying, J., et al. (2023). Incidence and Outcomes of Non–Ventilator-Associated Hospital-Acquired Pneumonia in 284 US Hospitals Using Electronic Surveillance Criteria. *JAMA Netw Open;6*(5):e2314185. https://jamanetwork.com/journals/jamanetworkopen/fullarticle/2805014

Shudaifat, Y., ALBashtawy, M., Qaddumi, J., Baqir, M., Zamzam, S., Ibnian, A., & Alkhawaldeh, A. (2021). The Role of Nursing Practice to Prevent Ventilator-associated Pneumonia in the Intensive Care Units. *Medico-Legal Update, 21*(3), 270–273. https://doi.org/10.37506/mlu.v21i3.2996

Kourtis, A. P., Hatfield, K., Baggs, J., Yi Mu, See, I., Epson, E.,

Nadle, J., Kainer, M. A., Dumyati, G., Petit, S., Ray, S. M., Ham, D., Capers, C., Ewing, H., Coffin, N., McDonald, L. C., Jernigan, J., Cardo, D., Mu, Y., & Emerging Infections Program MRSA author group (2019). Vital Signs: Epidemiology and Recent Trends in Methicillin-Resistant and in Methicillin-Susceptible Staphylococcus aureus Bloodstream Infections—United States. *Morbidity & Mortality Weekly Report, 68*(9), 214–219. https://doi.org/10.15585/mmwr.mm6809e1

Lee, B. Y., Bartsch, S. M., Wong, K. F., Singh, A., Avery, T. R., Kim, D. S., Brown, S. T., Murphy, C. R., Yilmaz, S. L., Potter, M. A., & Huang, S. S. (2013). The importance of nursing homes in the spread of methicillin-resistant Staphylococcus aureus (MRSA) among hospitals. *Medical care, 51*(3), 205–215. https://journals.lww.com/lww-medicalcare/fulltext/2013/03000/the_importance_of_nursing_homes_in_the_spread_of.1.aspx

Roney, J., Whitley, B., Maples, J., Futrell, L., Stunkard, K., & Long, J. (2015). Modified early warning scoring (MEWS): Evaluating the evidence for tool inclusion of sepsis screening criteria and impact on mortality and failure to rescue. *Journal of Clinical Nursing, 24*(23-24), 3343–3354. https://doi.org/10.1111/jocn.12952

Markwart, R., Saito, H., Harder, T., Tomczyk, S., Cassini, A., Fleischmann-Struzek, C., Reichert, F., Eckmanns, T., & Allegranzi, B. (2020). Epidemiology and burden of sepsis acquired in hospitals and intensive care units: a systematic review and meta-analysis. *Intensive Care Medicine, 46*(8), 1536–1551. https://doi.org/10.1007/s00134-020-06106-2

Chapter 13

Newman-Toker, D. E., Wang, Z., Zhu, Y., Nassery, N., Saber Tehrani, A. S., Schaffer, A. C., Yu-Moe, C. W., Clemens, G. D., Fanai, M., & Siegal, D. (2020). Rate of diagnostic errors and serious misdiagnosis-related harms for major vascular events, infections, and cancers: toward a national incidence estimate using the "Big Three". *Diagnosis (Berlin, Germany), 8*(1), 67–84. https://doi.org/10.1515/dx-2019-0104

Giardina, T. D., Hunte, H., Hill, M. A., Heimlich, S. L., Singh, H., Smith, K. M. (2022). Defining Diagnostic Error: A Scoping Review to Assess the Impact of the National Academies' Report Improving Diagnosis in Health Care, *Journal of Patient Safety* (10). 1097/PTS.0000000000000999. https://journals.lww.com/journalpatientsafety/fulltext/2022/12000/defining_diagnostic_error__a_scoping_review_to.7.aspx

Verna, R., Velazquez, A. B., & Laposata, M. (2019). Reducing diagnostic errors worldwide through diagnostic management teams. *Annals of Laboratory Medicine, 39*(2), 121–124. https://doi.org/10.3343/alm.2019.39.2.121

Graber, M. L., Wachter, R. M., & Cassel, C. K. (2012). Bringing diagnosis into the quality and safety equations. *JAMA, 308*(12), 1211–1212. https://doi.org/10.1001/2012.jama.11913

Baartmans, M. C., Hooftman, J., Zwaan, L., van Schoten, S. M., Erwich, J. J. H. M., & Wagner, C. (2022). What Can We Learn From In-Depth Analysis of Human Errors Resulting in Diagnostic Errors in the Emergency Department: An Analysis of Serious Adverse Event Reports. *Journal of Patient Safety.* https://doi.org/10.1097/PTS.0000000000001007

Schlachter, L. (2017). *Malpractice: a neurosurgeon reveals how our healthcare system puts patients at risk.* Skyhorse Publishing; 1st edition.

Al-Khafaji, J., Townshend, R. F., Townsend, W., et al (2022). Checklists to reduce diagnostic error: a systematic review of the literature using a human factors framework. *BMJ Open*, 12:e058219. https://bmjopen.bmj.com/content/12/4/e058219

Chapter 14

Al Khawaldeh, T. A., & Wazaify, M. (2018). Intravenous cancer chemotherapy administration errors: an observational study at referral hospital in Jordan. *European Journal of Cancer Care, 27*(4). https://doi.org/10.1111/ecc.12863

Caglar, D., & Kwum, R. (2011). Pediatric procedural sedation and analgesia in the emergency department. *Emergency Medicine Reports, 32*(18), 93–104.

Ragan, A. P., Aikens, G. B., Bounthavong, M., Brittain, K., & Mirk, A. (2021). Academic detailing to reduce sedative-hypnotic prescribing in older veterans. *Journal of Pharmacy Practice, 34*(2), 287–294. https://doi.org/10.1177/08971900 19870949

Hatatet, W., & Oakley, S. (2019). Nurses self-reporting and impression of compliance to chemotherapy administration safety standards and patient assessments: a multi-institute survey of oncology nurses in the Emirate of Abu Dhabi. *The Australian Journal of Cancer Nursing, 20*(1), 25–32. https://search.informit.org/doi/10.3316/informit.431079494875043

Sorrell, J. (2017). Ethics: ethical issues with medical errors: shaping a culture of safety in healthcare. *Ojin: The Online Journal of Issues in Nursing, 22*(2). https://doi.org/10.3912/OJIN.Vol22No02EthCol01

Chapter 15

Fernald, D. H., Pace, W. D., Harris, D. M., West, D. R., Main, D. S., Westfall, J. M. (2004). Event reporting to a primary care patient safety reporting system: a report from the ASIPS collaborative. *Ann Fam Med.2*(4):327–332.

Mohammad, A. A., Davari, F., Mansouri, M., Mohammadnia, M. (2017). Analysis of medical errors: a case study. *Med Ethics J. 10*(38):59–68.

Dimova, R., Stoyanova, R., & Doykov, I. (2018). Mixed-methods study of reported clinical cases of undesirable events, medical errors, and near misses in health care. *Journal of*

Evaluation in Clinical Practice, 24(4), 752–757. https://doi.org/10.1111/jep.12970

Patel, T. K., Patel, P. B., Bhalla, H. L., & Kishore, S. (2022). Drug-related deaths among inpatients: a meta-analysis. *European Journal of Clinical Pharmacology, 78*(2), 267–278. https://doi.org/10.1007/s00228-021-03214-w

Millenson, M. L. (2002). Pushing the profession: how the news media turned patient safety into a priority. *Quality in Health Care, 11*(1), 57–63.

Hodkinson, A., Tyler, N., Ashcroft, D. M., Keers, R. N., Khan, K., Phipps, D., Abuzour, A., Bower, P., Avery, A., Campbell, S., & Panagioti, M. (2020). Preventable medication harm across health care settings: a systematic review and meta-analysis. *Bmc Medicine, 18*(1), 313–313. https://doi.org/10.1186/s12916-020-01774-9

Bourne, R. S., Jeffries, M., Phipps, D. L., et al. (2023). Understanding medication safety involving patient transfer from intensive care to hospital ward: a qualitative sociotechnical factor study. *BMJ Open; 13*(5):e066757. http://dx.doi.org/10.1136/bmjopen-2022-066757

Chapter 16

American Association of Critical Care Nurses (AACN) (2018). More than half of enteral feeding tube misplacements were serious events. *AACN Bold Voices, April 1, pg. 11.* Retrieved from: https://www.aacn.org/education/publications/bold-voices/archive

Wallace, S. C. & Gardner, L. A. (2015). Misplacements of Enteral Feeding Tubes Increase After Hospitals Switch Brands. *AJN, American Journal of Nursing, 115* (8), 44–46. https://journals.lww.com/ajnonline/fulltext/2015/08000/misplacements_of_enteral_feeding_tubes_increase.24.aspx

ECRI (Emergency Care Research Institute) (2018). Top 10 Health Technology Hazards for 2018. https://www.ecri.org/Resources/Whitepapers_and_reports/Haz_18.pdf

Motta, A., Rigobello, M., Silveira, R., & Gimenes, F. (2021). Nasogastric/nasoenteric tube-related adverse events: an integrative review. Revista latino-americana de enfermagem, 29, e3400. https://doi.org/10.1590/1518-8345. 3355.3400

Wu. P. Y., Kang, T. J., Hui, C. K., Hung, M. H., Sun, W. Z., & Chan, W. H. (2006). Fatal Massive Hemorrhage Caused by Nasogastric Tube Misplacement in a Patient with Mediastinitis. *Journal of the Formosan Medical Association,* *105*(1), 80–85. https://doi.org/10.1016/S0929-6646(09)60113-3

Denver, M. A. S. G. (2009). A prospective multicenter evaluation of prehospital airway management performance in a large metropolitan region. *Prehospital Emergency Care,* *13*(3), 304–310. https://doi.org/10.1080/10903120902935280

Gnugnoli, D. M., Singh, A., Shafer, K. (2023). EMS Field Intubation In: StatPearls [Internet]. Treasure Island (FL): *StatPearls Publishing; 2023* Jan-. Available from: https:// www.ncbi.nlm.nih.gov/books/NBK538221/

Seyma, Z. K., Meral, Y. C., & Atiye, E. (2021). Nurses' Knowledge Levels About the Care of the Patients with Chest Tube. *International Journal of Caring Sciences, 14*(2), 1334–1342.

Kamio, T., Iizuka, Y., Koyama, H., & Fukaguchi, K. (2022). Adverse events related to thoracentesis and chest tube insertion: evaluation of the national collection of subject safety incidents in Japan. *European Journal of Trauma & Emergency Surgery, 48*(2), 981–988. https://doi.org/10.1007/ s00068-020-01575-y

Chapter 17

Jones, K. (2014). Alarm fatigue a top patient safety hazard: CMAJ. *Canadian Medical Association Journal, 186*(3), 178.

Ruppel, H., Funk, M., & Whittemore, R. (2018). Measurement of physiological monitor alarm accuracy and clinical relevance in intensive care units. *American Journal of*

Critical Care: An Official Publication, *American Association of Critical-Care Nurses, 27*(1), 11–21. https://doi.org/10.4037/ajcc2018385

Lewandowska, K., Weisbrot, M., Cieloszyk, A., Mędrzycka-Dąbrowska, W., Krupa, S., & Ozga, D. (2020). Impact of Alarm Fatigue on the Work of Nurses in an Intensive Care Environment-A Systematic Review. *International journal of environmental research and public health, 17*(22), 8409. https://doi.org/10.3390/ijerph17228409

Wong, M. (2014). Making the case for maximum alarm management and prevention of alarm fatigue. https://ppahs.org/2014/01/making-the-case-for-maximum-alarm-management-and-prevention-of-alarm-fatigue/

Graham, K. C., & Cvach, M. (2010). Monitor alarm fatigue: standardizing use of physiological monitors and decreasing nuisance alarms. *American Journal of Critical Care : an official publication, American Association of Critical-Care Nurses, 19*(1), 28–35. https://doi.org/10.4037/ajcc2010651

Chapter 18

Levinson, D. & Department of Health and Human Services (2010). Adverse event in Hospitals: National Incidence among Medicare Beneficiaries. OEI-06-09-00090 (Washington, CD: Office of the Inspector General.) https://oig.hhs.gov/oei/reports/oei-06-09-00090.pdf

Zaitoun, R. A., Said, N. B. & de Tantillo, L. (2023). Clinical nurse competence and its effect on patient safety culture: a systematic review. *BMC Nurs 22*, 173. https://doi.org/10.1186/s12912-023-01305-w

Crawford, C. L., Rondinelli, J., Zuniga, S., Valdez, R. M., Cullen, L., Hanrahan, K., & Titler, M. G. (2020). Testing of the nursing evidence-based practice survey. *Worldviews on Evidence-Based Nursing, 17*(2), 118–128. https://doi.org/10.1111/wvn.12432

Callen, J., Georgiou, A., Li, J., Westbrook, J. I. (2011). The safety

implications of missed test results for hospitalised patients:
a systematic review. *BMJ Qual Safety, 20*(2):194–9. Epub
2011 Feb 7. PMID: 21300992; PMCID: PMC3038104. https://
qualitysafety.bmj.com/content/20/2/194

Watson, B., Salmoni, A., & Zecevic, A. (2019). Case analysis
of factors contributing to patient falls. *Clinical Nursing
Research, 28*(8), 911–930. https://doi.org/10.1177/105477
3818754450

Fleisher, L. A., Schreiber, M., Cardo, D., & Srinivasan, A. (2022).
Health Care Safety during the Pandemic and Beyond—
Building a System That Ensures Resilience. *The New
England Journal of Medicine, 386*(7), 609–611. https://doi.
org/10.1056/NEJMp2118285

Borojeny, L., Albatineh, A., Dehkordi, A., & Gheshlagh, R.
(2020). The incidence of pressure ulcers and its associations
in different wards of the hospital: a systematic review and
meta-analysis. *International Journal of Preventive Medicine,
11*(1), 171–171. https://pubmed.ncbi.nlm.nih.gov/33312480/

Taylor, C., Mulligan, K., & McGraw, C. (2021). Barriers and
enablers to the implementation of evidence-based practice
in pressure ulcer prevention and management in an
integrated community care setting: A qualitative study
informed by the theoretical domains framework. *Health &
Social Care in the Community, 29*(3), 766–779. https://doi.
org/10.1111/hsc.13322

Chapter 19

Bonney, W. (2014). Medical errors: moral and ethical considerations. *J Hosp Adm, 32*(32), 80–88.

Verillo, S. C., & Winters, B. D. (2018). Review: Continuous
Monitoring to Detect Failure to Rescue in Adult
Postoperative Inpatients. *Biomedical Instrumentation &
Technology, 52*(4), 281–287. https://doi-org.chamberlain
university.idm.oclc.org/10.2345/0899-8205-52.4.281

Cohen, A. J., Lui, H., Zheng, M., Cheema, B., Patino, G., Kohn, M. A., Enriquez, A., & Breyer, B. N. (2021). Rates of serious surgical errors in California and plans to prevent recurrence. *Jama Network Open, 4*(5), 217058. https://doi.org/10.1001/jamanetworkopen.2021.7058

Anderson, O., Davis, R., Hanna, G. B., Vincent, C. A. (2013). Surgical adverse events: a systematic review. *Am J Surg, 206*(2), 253–62. Epub 2013 May 1. PMID: 23642651. https://doi.org/10.1016/j.amjsurg.2012.11.009

Thiels, C. A., Lal, T. M., Nienow, J. M., Pasupathy, K. S., Blocker, R. C., Aho, J. M., . . . Bingener, J. (2015). Surgical never events and contributing human factors. *Surgery,158,* 515–21. http://dx.doi.org/10.1016/j.surg.2015.03.053

Landers, R. (2015). Reducing Surgical Errors: Implementing a Three-Hinge Approach to Success: The Official Voice of Perioperative Nursing. *AORN Journal, 101*(6), 657–665. https://doi.org/10.1016/j.aorn.2015.04.013

Peponis, T., Baekgaard, J. S., Bohnen, J. D., Han, K., Lee, J., Saillant, N., Fagenholz, P., King, D. R., Velmahos, G. C., Kaafarani, H. M. A. (2018). Are surgeons reluctant to accurately report intraoperative adverse events? A prospective study of 1,989 patients. *Surgery, 164*(3):525–529. Epub 2018 Jun 24. PMID: 29945783. https://doi.org/10.1016/j.surg.2018.04.035

De Cassai, A., Negro, S., Geraldini, F., Boscolo, A., Sella, N., Munari, M., Navalesi, P., & Mordaunt, D. A. (2021). Inattentional blindness in anesthesiology: a gorilla is worth one thousand words. *Plos One, 16*(9). https://doi.org/10.1371/journal.pone.0257508

Omar, I., Singhal, R., Wilson, M., Parmar, C., Khan, O., & Mahawar, K. (2021). Sp7.1.5 common general surgical never events: analysis of nhs england never events data. *British Journal of Surgery,* 108(Supplement 7). https://doi.org/10.1093/bjs/znab361.141

Verma, A., Tran, Z., Hadaya, J., Williamson, C. G., Rahimtoola, R., & Benharash, P. (2021). Factors Associated With Retained Foreign Bodies Following Major Operations. *The American Surgeon, 87*(10), 1575–1579. https://doi. org/10.1177/00031348211024969

Harris, K., Søfteland, E., Moi, A. L., Harthug, S., Storesund, A., Jesuthasan, S., . . . Haugen, A. S. (2020). Patients' and healthcare workers' recommendations for a surgical patient safety checklist—a qualitative study. *England: BioMed Central.* https://doi.org/10.1186/s12913-020-4888-1

Ferraris, V. A., Bolanos, M., Martin, J. T., Mahan, A., & Saha, S. P. (2014). Identification of patients with postoperative complications who are at risk for failure to rescue. *Jama Surgery, 149*(11), 1103–8. https://doi.org/10.1001/jamasurg. 2014.1338

Caparelli, M. L., Shikhman, A., Jalal, A., Oppelt, S., Ogg, C., & Allamaneni, S. (2019). Prevention of postoperative pneumonia in noncardiac surgical patients: a prospective study using the national surgical quality improvement program database. *The American Surgeon, 85*(1), 8–14.

Abboud, J., Abdel Rahman, A., Kahale, L., Dempster, M., & Adair, P. (2020). Prevention of health care associated venous thromboembolism through implementing vte prevention clinical practice guidelines in hospitalized medical patients: a systematic review and meta-analysis. *Implementation Science Is, 15*(1), 49–49. https://doi.org/10.1186/s13012-020-01008-9

Maynard, G. (2015). *Preventing hospital-associated venous thromboembolism: a guide for effective quality improvement,* 2nd ed. Rockville, MD: Agency for Healthcare Research and Quality; October 2015. AHRQ Publication No. 16-0001-EF.

Krauss, B., & Green, S. M. (2008). Training and credentialing in procedural sedation and analgesia in children: lessons from the United States model. *Pediatric Anesthesia, 18*(1), 30–35. https://doi.org/10.1111/j.1460-9592.2007.02406.x

Hixenbaugh, M. (2019). No one should die from a blood transfusion. So why did it happen at MD Anderson, the nation's top cancer hospital? https://www.nbcnews.com/news/us-news/no-one-should-die-blood-transfusion-so-why-did-it-n1021506

Conclusion

Bates, D. W., Levine, D. M., Salmasian, H., Syrowatka, A., Shahian, D. M., Lipsitz, S., Zebrowski, J. P., Myers, L. C., Logan, M. S., Roy, C. G., Iannaccone, C., Frits, M. L., Volk, L. A., Dulgarian, S., Amato, M. G., Edrees, H. H., Sato, L., Folcarelli, P., Einbinder, J. S., . . . Mort, E. (2023). The safety of inpatient health care. *The New England Journal of Medicine, 388*(2), 142–153. https://doi.org/10.1056/NEJMsa2206117

Ahsani-Estahbanati E, Sergeevich Gordeev V., & Doshmangir L. (2022). Interventions to reduce the incidence of medical error and its financial burden in health care systems: A systematic review of systematic reviews. *Front. Med.* 9:875426. https://doi.org/10.3389/fmed.2022.875426

Fleisher, L. A., Schreiber, M., Cardo, D., & Srinivasan, A. (2022). Health Care Safety during the Pandemic and Beyond—Building a System That Ensures Resilience. *The New England Journal of Medicine, 386*(7), 609–611. https://doi.org/10.1056/NEJMp2118285

ABOUT THE AUTHOR

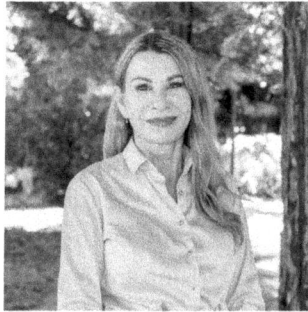

Dr. Julie Siemers brings more than four decades of experience and expertise in nursing practice, education, and executive leadership to the healthcare arena. Dr. Siemers direct patient care experience includes a wide variety of roles on the medical/surgical care floor, Intensive Care Unit, emergency department, and trauma resuscitation department at University Medical Center, Las Vegas. She has served as Chief Flight Nurse and Regional Program Director for Mercy Air Services in Las Vegas. Dr. Siemers is passionate about education in healthcare; she served as an education consultant and Account Executive for a large medical device company for several years and was instrumental in impacting positive changes in patient monitoring practices. Dr. Siemers has been a member of State Boards of Nursing Education Councils to contribute her expertise to enhancing safe nursing practice.

Dr. Siemers' has been a great influence in nursing education for the past fourteen years serving in various capacities of Professor of Nursing for Adult Health and Critical Care courses, Program Director of the Bachelor of Science in Nursing at Touro

University, Dean of Academic Affairs, Campus President in Arlington Virginia and Jacksonville Florida for Chamberlain University. Current and future nurses need to be vigilant in their practice and care of patients to improve patient outcomes and save lives. Dr. Siemers currently serves as Campus Executive Director for a large Nursing University in California and is responsible for providing strategic direction to successfully achieve academic and operational goals—building upon past successes and driving excellence in nursing education.

Dr. Siemers earned a Master of Science in Nursing and Doctor of Nursing Practice degrees from Touro University, Nevada. Dr. Siemers graduate and doctoral projects were centered around her passion for patient safety and the urgent necessity of creating substantial and sustainable changes in current healthcare practice. Dr. Siemers focus and vision for creating radical changes in healthcare to protect patients from unintended harm and preventable medical errors is to inform and educate each and every patient and their family members. To be forewarned is to be forearmed. We are all in this together.

To learn more or to contact Dr. Siemers visit
www.DrJulieSiemers.com

www.ingramcontent.com/pod-product-compliance
Lightning Source LLC
Chambersburg PA
CBHW072339090426
42741CB00012B/2842

9 789898 628301 2